MW00876463

Bariatric Mindset Success
Live Your Best Life and Keep the Weight Off After Weight Loss Surgery

Kristin Lloyd, PhD

Bariatric Mindset Success

Copyright © 2017 by Kristin Lloyd

Note from the publisher: The authors and publisher of this book disclaim all liability in connection with the use of this book, and disavow all knowledge of personal details written into this after publication. The contents of this book are solely for the purchaser's private use and will be treated as such under the jurisdiction of the United States of America, and under recognized international publishing laws. All persons concerned about medical symptoms or the possibility of disease are encouraged to seek professional care from an appropriate health-care provider.

NOTE: We are grateful to clients for allowing us to share personal details from their lives. Due to medical privacy laws (HIPAA), names, dates, ages, and locations may have been changed to protect identities. Any similarity to actual persons is purely coincidental. In no way is this book designed to replace, substitute, countermand, or conflict with advice given to you by your physician, or mental health professional. Information in this book is offered with no guarantees on the part of the authors or publisher. Mention of specific individuals, companies, organizations, or authorities in this book does not imply endorsement by the authors or publisher.

This book is not intended as a substitute for the medical advice of physicians. The reader should regularly consult a physician in matters relating to his/her health and particularly with respect to any symptoms that may require diagnosis or medical attention. While the author is a licensed counseling professional, the recommendations or suggestions contained in this book are based on her personal and professional experiences dealing with bariatrics. The author attempted to recreate events, locales, and conversations from her memories of them. In order to maintain anonymity, names of individuals have been changed.

Printed in the United States of America
First Printing, 2017

Cover Design by Ascent Graphics & Design, Inc.

Dedication

For most of my life, I felt "not good enough." I attracted all the wrong people into my life, and I knew I needed to make a change within myself. I began on a path toward self-love, recognizing that to attract love, I had to love me first. It was then that my "good enough" was reflected by someone who loved me as is. My husband is the man who saw me for me, by loving me at 330 lb. when we first met, 340 lb. when we married, at over 400 lb. after our first child, and now after all my weight loss. He loved me fat, he loved me thin, the truth is he has always loved me from within.

He has shown me the most love, compassion, and called me out on my excuses. He's been my biggest cheerleader, my rock, and the one who helped me not give up on myself when the going got tough. Therefore, I dedicate this book to him. I love you Hobb – you're my everything.

To my son, who was our surprise pregnancy when I originally tried to get bariatric surgery in 2012. He was the showstopper that year. It's because of you both, that I decided to recommit myself to my health. So much so that I decided to have bariatric surgery, which inevitably changed my life forever. That step led me to my purpose of helping others on a similar journey.

Preface

The decision to have bariatric surgery is one of the most important decisions that anyone will make in his or her life. There are hundreds of people who make this decision daily, and it is important to make sure there's a clear path to the finish line for them. Many of the books available focus on what to eat, how much to eat, and what to expect after bariatric surgery.

In this book, I go beyond the food. I focus on trying to lay out the path of the physical, spiritual, and the mental/emotional processes. This is to ensure that every patient has a way to know that he or she will be taken care of and that they will make their journey with someone who has taken the journey herself.

There is nothing more important than understanding the day-to-day issues that are also a part of the experience. I am going to walk you through this journey as a person who has had bariatric surgery, who has experienced both the highs and the lows, and as a professional who can help you overcome your inner saboteur and rebuild your mindset in the process leading you to your most successful, and skinny, self.

Acknowledgments

A special thanks to my girlfriends LC Taylor of LC Taylor Publishings and Crystal Jones Harrison of Ascent Graphics and Design, Inc. Without the two of you, this book would not have been published on time!

But a special thanks to all my bariatric clients. This book would not be possible had you not believed in yourselves to do the necessary work, all while putting your faith in me as your counselor and coach, giving me the opportunity to guide you to greatness!

Table of Contents

COPYRIGHT II

DEDICATION III

PREFACE IV

ACKNOWLEDGMENTS V

INTRODUCTION 1

CHAPTER 1 8

   My Story 9

   Cravings vs Emotional Eating 15

   Breaking Free of Victim Mentality or Victim Cycle 17

   Stress, Anxiety & Discouragement 19

   The Reinforcement of "Not Enough" 20

   Poor Emotional Boundaries 22

   Settling vs Being Comfortable 24

   The Elephant in the Room 25

   Building Awareness is the First Step 27

CHAPTER 2 31

   Bariatric Surgery and Nutrition 38

   Protein 42

   Vegetables 43

   Liquids 44

   Supplements 47

   Avoid Slider Foods & Grazing 48

   Other Basic Elements for Your Weight Loss Success 49

   The Therapeutic Component 51

   Exercise 54

   Busting Up Excuses 60

   Starting Your Exercise Program 62

   Your New Mindset After the Honeymoon is Over 63

   Chapter Review and Exercises 67

   Important Elements 68

CHAPTER 3 69

   Goal Setting Basics 73

Visualize the Outcome You Desire 81

Past/Future Self – Creating a Plan...89

Meal Planning..92

Exercise Planning..96

Stopping the "Do It Tomorrow" Attitude...99

Emotional Struggle with "Not Doing Things" Procrastination and Fear of Success / Fear of Failure 102

Chapter Journaling Prompts 109

CHAPTER 4 110

Building Consistency = Creating New Behaviors & Habits.......................119

Creating Motivation 122

Cultivating Success through Perseverance 129

CHAPTER 5 131

Your Support System and Asking for Help 132

CHAPTER 6 143

Eating Mindfully 144

Exercise 1: Mindful Eating 146

Exercise 2: Conscious Eating..148

EFT..151

What's the Process? How Do I Do It? 153

Tapping Scripts 156

MBSR (Mindfulness-Based Stress Reduction) 159

Progressive Muscle Relaxation 163

Visualization Exercises...165

Journaling 168

Journaling Exercises..171

Food and Feelings: How to Recognize and Address Emotional Eating 174

Identifying Healthy Behaviors for Your Growth.......................................180

CHAPTER 7 183

History, Causes & the Theory of Eating Behaviors...................................190

Getting off the Emotional Eating Rollercoaster.......................................192

Digging Deeper, Slowing Down, & Being Conscious 196

How Do I Measure Something I Cannot Name and Always Avoid?.........202

E3 – Exercise, Excuses, and Your Emotions..205

Compassion ≠ Permission or Self-Indulgence 208

The Controversial Topic of Self-Love *211*

Remember Your Visualizations: Your Photo Album for the Future *220*

CHAPTER 8 .... *224*

Friendships: Dealing with Jealousy, Anger, and Other Issues *225*

Romantic Relationships *228*

For the Already Married WLS Patient: How to Maintain or Improve Your
Marriage *234*

Five Ways People Can Navigate Relationships through the Ins and Outs of
Life after Bariatric Surgery *239*

Celebrate Success with Your Partner *244*

Setting Healthy Boundaries *245*

Sex and Sexual Advances after WLS *257*

CHAPTER 9 .... *260*

Effects of Emergency Mode *266*

CHAPTER 10 .... *269*

Building Your Bucket List *276*

Affirming Your Dreams *279*

APPENDICES *286*

BIBLIOGRAPHY *290*

ABOUT THE AUTHOR *293*

Introduction

It was a Tuesday.

I remember it as clear as though it was yesterday. It was the summer of 2010; I was in my office sitting with new clients. I was sitting in the burnt sienna colored armchair, fidgeting with my pen and clipboard, reading over the client's intake packet.

My clients were a couple who were there for their first session, and I was worried I wouldn't make a good impression. I remember distinctly we were discussing the wife's yoga routine, as it was pertinent to some of the issues coming up in their marriage. Nothing they brought to the session triggered me, or in my mind, brought up "transference" or "countertransference" in therapy terms.

However, in my mind, my negative inner critic was having a field day. The wife was a sprightly woman, about five feet eight inches and skinny as a rail. The husband was also very fit. Even though the topic of yoga and exercise came up, their issues had absolutely NOTHING to do with weight. Yet, somehow, I felt inadequate in my ability to help them in my current physical state at that time.

"You know they can see how fat you are! How can you possibly help them if you can't even help yourself?" My inner self shouted at me.

As a therapist and coach, I was well aware of negative self-talk and the inner critic that everyone has. Mine grew increasingly louder as time went on. This wasn't the first or last time, I would hear her voice in my head. It was the loudest time I remember, and the most potent it had been in a while.

I quickly pushed my thoughts to focus on my client's needs; however, it was in this moment, within my own head, I was judging myself. Later on, outside of the session, I reflected on what happened. I was horrified and terrified, about whether I was actually qualified to help others, purely due to my own fight with obesity.

Am I qualified? I thought to myself.

This inner angst was gnawing. Of course, I was. I'd done the schoolwork, finished my degree, completed the required internships, and was working on licensing hours under a qualified supervisor. Later, I took my thoughts to my supervisor in one of our sessions, because it bothered me so much.

I wasn't immune to how other people looked at me. I'm five feet eleven inches tall. I'm not a small person, and prior to surgery, my average daily weight was over 375 lb. (I typically went up and down like a yo-yo). In my mind, I resembled one of Seattle's best linebackers. Often times, I refused to get on the scale at the doctor's office because it would depress me, as if hiding from the scale would make the weight go away.

Although when I did weigh in, it was a reality check. I typically avoided seeing the "reality" because I would go into a shame spiral, causing my inner critic to squawk louder. I would wind up feeling like total and utter shit. From that moment on, I felt like a failure. This wouldn't get me rolling on the latest diet plan, instead, it would make me want to eat silently and in private – further perpetuating the cycle of obesity in my life.

Shame. Guilt. Fear. Doubt. Self-hatred and a complete lack of self-trust around food. I knew them well – I lived with them. They were my friends. They were my enemies.

The day I saw my highest weight was a day I'll never forget.

It was in early 2013, and I'd gone into urgent care – of course, they wanted to weigh me. The nurse put me on the scale, saying she needed it for my chart. I tried to refuse, but she told me it was policy and smiled. She was trying to be sweet and probably knew I was dying inside. She looked at me with loving eyes as though she knew it was no secret the number was going to be on the high side.

Somehow, I'd convinced myself if no one saw the number, it wouldn't be real. The moment is burned into my memory. I cringed, gasping when I saw it – 411 lb. The nurse was kind enough to not read it out loud in the hallway.

Instead, she said, "OK, honey, you can get down now, I've recorded it," tapping me on the arm. "It'll be OK."

But I started to get angry. Not with her, but with myself. How did I not know? How did I let it get this far? I couldn't believe my eyes. The rationalization started to kick in as she walked me to the procedure room.

Maybe their scale was off, I said to myself.

Clearly, this was all justification for my poor choices and emotional eating, which I consciously knew was out of control. I used to tell myself, and others, that I didn't eat much; however, once everyone went to bed, I'd sit with a huge bowl of ice cream, cleaning up the evidence afterward.

I remember crying after I left the doctor's office, not because of the weight itself, but at the enormity that I'd become. The truth was, I didn't really SEE myself, and when I did, I would make excuses saying, you're not THAT big.

It was like I had reverse body dysmorphia where in my mind I'd rationalized I just wasn't as big as I really was. I also hid from mirrors and from "seeing" myself, because I would not stand in front of a mirror for very long – if at all.

How did I let it get this far? How had I done this to myself? Those were the questions I asked over and over.

The truth was, this was not a one-time event. This was the one event that sticks out in my mind. Over the years, I familiarized myself with diet clinics, pills, plans, diets, exercise routines, prepackaged food, and so much more.

Dieting was a lifestyle I lived for way too long. It was paired with going off the diet when I experienced a binge due to a bad day, a good day, a celebration, or a binge for many other reasons. The truth that I hadn't figured out, until much later, was my emotions were tied to food – and I didn't know how to adjust or stop it.

As I flashback in my mind, even as a youngster, thoughts and feelings about food plagued my mind. Even now, I remember a moment that now registers as odd. In second grade, I had this pervasive nightmare.

In the nightmare, I would bust into the classroom while all the other students were at one of our extracurriculars, and one by one eat their lunch in the back of the room by the cubbyholes. I would see myself in the back of the classroom, lunchboxes sprawled out on the floor, emptied, and me, caught in the room alone as everyone comes to the door. I remember feeling shame and horror.

I don't remember it being about the food; however, I remember the feelings of shame and remorse from eating everyone else's food, leaving the other kids without anything to eat for lunch. This was a very persistent nightmare that replayed frequently in my mind.

I have no idea what put these thoughts in my head, nor did I recognize the connection to my food issues until much later in life. The focus of the dream was clearly centered around fear, shame for eating the food, being caught with food, and me having food that others did not have.

Often times I feared going to the playground because my younger brothers would shout that I was fat. I was mortified that others would see me in that light. Attending a parochial school, we all wore these strait-bodied, no curve showing uniforms. I realize now, looking back, I was not fat nor heavy. I might have been considered "thick"; however, the idea that I could be a "FAT GIRL," horrified me. The idea of being classified in that manner took up way too much space in my head.

These and many other similar situations have played a part in forming the central theme in my life. I've consistently dealt with issues centered around food – even after having bariatric surgery.

Yep, you read that correctly, even after bariatric surgery.

That's the main reason you are here reading this. Most people think bariatric surgery fixes all the issues. The truth is, it does NOT. It helps people to lose the weight by shrinking their stomach. What it does NOT do is help people deal with emotional food issues or food cravings that can still linger following surgery.

Bariatric surgery is a lifestyle change, and it is instrumental that people implement the mindset shifts necessary to sustain that long-term change. Otherwise, they'll rebound, returning to their original pre-surgery weight. It's sad but true, and I've witnessed this happen to countless others.

It's not always likely to happen, so don't scare yourself into oblivion. BUT, if you do not take the necessary life-changing steps aligning your mindset and emotional food issues after surgery, you risk regaining weight.

Chapter 1

Your Former Self

Who you were before bariatric surgery and who you are after, will be drastically different. You will change for the good, and there will be experiences and situations that stretch you emotionally and psychologically, while you are shrinking physically.

My life prior to bariatric surgery is completely different from life after bariatric surgery. In this chapter, I'll share with you parts of my journey as a bariatric patient and ask you to evaluate your own. This is also where you begin to see the differences in who you were and who you are going to become. This is a process, so don't feel that you must rush it. There will be ups and downs. There will be struggles and triumphs.

Knowing who you were prior to bariatric surgery is important to reflect on so that you have the awareness of that person, their thoughts, feelings/emotions, behaviors/actions, and who you want to become. This process is important for discovering who you were before surgery and who you want to become after surgery.

My Story

Like many people who take this path, I'd attempted just about everything under the sun to lose weight and keep it off. As you might imagine, much like your own journey, nothing worked for me. To add insult to injury, the diet and weight loss industry is a multi-billion-dollar empire. An empire that leaves many people feeling helpless and hopeless, with empty pockets and not much consistent weight loss to boot.

I would see a new advertisement, and getting my hopes up, I'd invest in the new product or service. Surely THIS would be the thing to FINALLY change my life and get the weight off. My life for a while seemed consumed with weight loss, weight loss activities, and dieting. Magazine covers are layered with images of perfect men and women. Even though they are most often photoshopped to appear perfect, these images continue to further this perfectionistic society's ideal of what people "should" look like.

I would look in the mirror – I was far from perfect. All I saw was a person I hated, trapped in a body that would not change. When it got too much for me to handle, the image in the mirror, I would do what many people in my situation would do: eat. I ate to soothe the negative feelings of disdain. For me this, in and of itself, felt like a sickness. The process would begin again – eating to rid myself of the negative feelings, and dieting, in an attempt to love myself again. It was a vicious cycle.

Another conclusion I reached during this time was if my life wasn't surrounded by and focused on attempting to lose weight, planning meals, and working out every day – then I was gaining weight. This would cause me to grow more discouraged.

I found myself asking myself, why bother?

This negative cycle I found myself perpetuating in led to one thing – me continuing to gain weight.

Does this sound familiar?

Over the course of my life, I tried traditional dieting, nontraditional dieting, purchased food plans (where they mail you the food), weight loss pills (both prescribed and over the counter), supplements, shakes, workout videos, gym memberships, hypnotherapy, doctor facilitated weight loss, personal trainers, nutritionists, Overeater's Anonymous (OA), and even a special eating disorders psychologist. In any given venture, I would lose 30–50 lb. (give or take), and then gain it all back.

None of these programs were sustainable for me or helped me focus on long-term change. They were all short-term fixes for a lifelong issue.

Looking back, I can even give a timeline.

In 2004–2008, phentermine was my best friend. Losing and gaining 30–50 lb. depending on whether I was on it or not.

In 2009, I was living abroad and lost weight naturally and arbitrarily because I walked to my job every day. When I moved back to the US later that year, I gained a significant amount of weight back.

In 2010, I had a personal trainer, a nutritionist, and probably tried multiple plans that year. I fought with food very hard in 2010. I remember hiding food and having periods of binging as well. I never purged, but the binging would be significant, eating whole pizzas at a time, and hiding the evidence.

From 2010 to 2011, I tried a generalized hypnotherapy. I went weekly, to sit in a chair where they put lights on my eyes and sent me home with hypnotherapy CDs to listen to twice a day. I was religious about listening to my CDs. My weight loss stalled.

In 2011, I realized that maybe my struggle was psychological in nature. I was convinced there was something wrong with me. There had to be!

I was stuck at 385 lb., and if I wasn't COMPLETELY focused on losing weight, I was gaining weight. My life had become all about food. I was disgusted and frustrated feeling like I was in prison.

Fed up, I made a decision … I decided to see an eating disorders psychologist – hoping it would be the answer and my savior. I found someone who had a long list of credentials and experience in dealing with people who had eating disorders. What happened next shocked and frustrated me beyond belief.

The eating disorder's psychologist experience I had was extremely frustrating because she wanted to focus on my food intake. I tried to be patient, but by session four she was still focused on what I was eating.

At this point, I'd become extremely frustrated because I was ready to dig into the emotional stuff. I was ready to talk about my family, my friends, my poor choices, my behaviors, and the emotions. I wasn't hiding the food or my poor habits, and in fact, I wanted to talk about them.

I was ready! I wanted to discuss how awful I felt, why I ate, when I ate, how much I ate, and the reasons I ate. I was ready to dig deep! However, what happened frustrated me the most; she wanted to discuss the food and only the food. I'd realized without her, it wasn't about the food, it was about my feelings. So, by session eight, I quit. I wasn't getting what I knew I needed, even after asking for what I felt I needed from her and our work together. She was still hyper-focused on the food.

The biggest realization I've had from my journey prior to bariatric surgery, and then after bariatric surgery, is this:

Most people tend to focus on the food, but it's not actually about the food. It's about the feelings hidden beneath the surface that go unnoticed. It's about the emotions that don't get felt, because they're covered by the urge to eat, the need to self-soothe, and the need to avoid the feelings altogether.

Food was my coping mechanism. I ate to push down the feelings I didn't want to feel. Regardless, I couldn't see this in myself, and no therapist I saw, could see this either. I'd visited many people regarding my food and eating issues, hoping that I'd be set free from my poor habits and lose the weight once and for all.

Yet each time, I'd have someone discuss dieting and the food. They would try putting me on a diet, making the food the central issue again. They would try to normalize the food and make me feel better. Yet, instead, it made me feel like I had a horrible affliction.

I share this story today, to let you know these feelings are normal, and there is NOTHING wrong with you. Many people struggle with these same issues, and that's why I'm sharing this with you in this book.

In my own journey, and as a clinician working with others on a similar journey, I've realized that the food was not the central issue. Instead, it was a symptom of much deeper emotional issues.

It was after bariatric surgery that this belief was further confirmed. I remember eating dinner with my family, my pouch was comfortably full. My emotional/mental self still wanted food, yet my physical self (my pouch / smaller stomach) would not allow it.

This was both a blessing and a curse. This is what I'd always wanted. Yet, the emotional side of me wasn't satisfied, when my physical body was. This is likely what you'll experience, or may have already experienced depending on where you are in your journey.

Cravings vs Emotional Eating

In my work as a clinician, I've seen things within my patients that are normal for individuals struggling with obesity. I've found a list of typical behaviors, emotions, and belief systems, many of my clients identify with. This is not a complete list; however, these are the most common ones I've encountered in my experience and professional practice with bariatric patients.

There are two things to be aware of: cravings and emotional eating.

They're different.

A craving is when you want a specific food. Cravings can be due to a couple of things. For example, sometimes our bodies crave chocolate due to low magnesium.

Other times it's because our over time our brains become wired neurologically to think that chocolate tastes good, and we desire chocolate because of how it tastes.

Emotional eating, however, is a bit different.

Emotional eating is the need to stuff something in your mouth because of how you feel. Typically, you're not focused on what you are eating, as long as you are eating. Emotional eating happens as a response to an emotion. When I was asked to start producing YouTube videos for Bariatric Mindset, I was aware I felt anxious and tense.

I reflected and recognized that all I wanted to do at that moment was shove food, any kind of food, in my mouth to relieve the tension. It was an "aha" moment for me as I realized anxiety was a trigger for emotional eating. Thankfully, I was self-aware enough at the time, and I have a toolbox full of activities to call on to pull me out of that space; however, for many, the emotional triggers cause people to overeat.

Building awareness of your eating behaviors is critical to help you recognize if you struggle with emotional eating. Everyone is different, and each person will not have the same emotional response to food.

When building self-awareness, it's important you create a list of coping mechanisms or other tools to utilize instead of eating. This will help you soothe your feelings and bring you out of the negative emotional state you're experiencing. You will learn to use a more appropriate response to your feelings rather than using food.

Breaking Free of Victim Mentality or Victim Cycle

Like emotional eating, there are individuals within the obesity community who do not take personal responsibility for their actions. I can tell you first and foremost that no one shoved food down my throat or carried me through countless drive-throughs.

That was ALL me.

However, I still felt like a victim of my own issues. Likewise, many of my clients feel out of control with food, and struggle with the idea of "never eating this or that again." This process is not about deprivation or not eating a certain food ever again. Instead, it's about being wise with your choices, and taking personal responsibility for those choices.

As someone who tipped the scales at over 400 lb., I know there were times when I was in full-on victim mode, blaming external factors for my own emotional responses. I see where the excuses become rampant when someone feels the struggle, or is unwilling to act in their lives.

Having weight loss surgery is the first step in breaking out of the victim cycle because this means you are acting and doing something to take back control over yourself and your life.

The steps after that are action-based. You'll need to get up and walk. You'll need to make food that is nourishing for your body. You'll need to eat when physically hungry, not when you're emotionally hungry. As I stated above, the emotional hunger or head hunger will be around for a while.

It's through the mindset work, you begin to build the muscles within your mind to break the chains of the psychological/emotional need to eat. Eating to soothe is a habit and breaking free from that takes commitment and consistency. You would not walk into a gym once and expect to look like a bodybuilder; the same is true for transforming your mindset and releasing the emotional need for food.

Breaking out of the victim mentality, or victim cycle, is about taking back control over your choices and taking a stand for yourself. This is your life, and bariatric surgery was likely the key to saving you from yourself and your past poor choices. As someone who has been down that road, I empathize and recognize that there is no time to live in the past. When you do, you can often get stuck there.

The step you have taken to have bariatric surgery is your future. You must look to the future and do something different, so you do not repeat the past or go back and live there. It's time that you take back control over your life for good and start living with yourself in the driver's seat.

Stress, Anxiety & Discouragement

Stress, anxiety, and discouragement are emotions that can trigger your feelings of "not enough."

Stress is your body's response to pressure or a threat. Stress is an issue when it comes to obesity because it triggers adrenaline and cortisol production during times that are filled with tension. Stress, anxiety, and discouragement can turn overeating into a habit and a coping mechanism. Over time, stress can build up and turn into anxiety, causing cortisol to be produced regularly, which leads to an increase in weight.

Additionally, the cycle of emotions repeats when stress and anxiety are present over and over. It can be discouraging when someone does everything they know, to lose the weight, and not much weight is lost. Over time the discouragement leads to a return of old habits, and from a psychological perspective, the person may resort to "giving up" because they feel they've worked so hard for such little result.

We'll work on how to reduce your stress levels, and also look at how you can manage and master your stress, so you can continue to lose the weight – no matter what. Having adequate tools in your toolbox to combat stress is what you'll need to conquer stress and keep the weight off.

The Reinforcement of "Not Enough"

Not Good Enough …

Not Thin Enough …

Not Pretty Enough …

Not Smart Enough …

Not _____ Enough …

This is what I call the plague of "not enough."

From an emotional standpoint, this can be created in childhood or in young adulthood, as individuals compare themselves to what they "should" look like, who they "should" be, and so on.

The syndrome of "not enough" also keeps people from reaching their highest potential, because this stimulates the idea of "why bother?" The cycle of emotions repeats itself, and the individual struggling with obesity gives up. They don't believe they'll ever reach the goals they've set for themselves because the bar is set so high in their own minds.

It's important, however, that this "not enough" differs from victim mentality or having poor boundaries. When individuals see themselves as not measuring up and being "not enough," what happens is they stop striving to be their best selves. This is because they believe, inherently at their very core, that no matter what, they won't level up or measure up to the comparison. Therefore, the self-sabotage ensues instead of trying to be the best person they can be and dealing with their own emotions.

When individuals fail to process emotions while going through the cycle of "not enough," they tend to avoid the feelings because it hurts so much. As a result, they do not feel the feelings and numb themselves instead. In the case of obesity, typically with food, this continues the cycle of not feeling good enough, the eating leads to weight gain, furthering the belief that they'll never measure up.

Poor Emotional Boundaries

Long before I started working with individuals struggling with obesity, I found myself in a conundrum of sorts. I would have a hard time telling people "NO" and ended up taking on more than I could handle. Then, in situations where I had to say "no" because I just couldn't, I would apologize constantly for not being able to meet everyone's needs. As a result, from trying to be that girl that wants everyone to like her, I ended up being the girl that no one respected. This was one of those things I did to myself and realized it once I started on my path following bariatric surgery.

I've seen it in my clients too. Mary always said "yes" at work and desired the praise. Amanda said "yes" to her family, and, as a result, lost the respect of her children. Amy wanted everyone to like her, so she went out of her way to do everything for everyone else, and, as a result, had no time for herself.

Michael wanted to be seen and heard, so he took on work from his boss he was never paid for or acknowledged for, and it left him feeling overwhelmed and used. There are a dozen more examples of individuals who couldn't say "no," due to fear of what others would say to them, about them, or fear of being judged in general.

The truth is, when you set boundaries, emotional or otherwise, you're taking a stand for yourself. Poor boundaries with friends, family, colleagues, and in other relationships don't get you liked. In fact, they do the opposite.

You tend to lose friends, family, and other relationships. In the long run, you end up resentful of how much your relationships are costing you. Relationships are meant to be reciprocal, and if you are allowing others to step all over you, this is not a reciprocal relationship.

Take a look into your own life and relationships, and evaluate where you continually say "YES," despite your best intentions. We will also work on how to set better boundaries, and gain the respect of your colleagues, family, and friends ... so you have happier and healthier relationships.

Settling vs Being Comfortable

Settling for less than one deserves is something my clients unanimously agree that they do. Sometimes they think they are doing things that make them "comfortable"; however, when we dig deeper below the surface, they are typically settling because of the fear of rejection, too much work, or again, the plague of "I'm not yet enough."

People settle for mediocrity in many aspects of their lives daily, out of fear. Usually, it doesn't pop up as fear but might show up as inadequacy, doubt, shame, or in the form of "not good enough" type thinking.

People settle for the jobs they hate, the friends or relationships that they may not get the most from, or deal with people letting them down all the time. They settle for what they think they can "get," instead of going after what they really want. The truth is, this goes way deeper than obesity, and the practice of settling has been going on a while.

You know it and I know it.

The former you would continue to settle, while the new vibrant you is busting to get out. As we move forward in this book, we'll go beyond settling. Allowing you to reach for what you truly desire in life, so you can stop living at life's most basic level.

It's time for you to rise out of mediocrity and take a stand to "never settle" in any area of your life.

The Elephant in the Room

Get off the "Weight" Cycle – Stop Focusing on the Weight.

So many people think their weight is about the weight. Once I had bariatric surgery and started losing the weight, I recognized how my weight was not about the weight at all. This is the part where you may become emotionally challenged because you will begin to question all the things that you haven't before.

✓ Who are you?

✓ Who are you really?

✓ What do you really want for your life?

What is stopping you from living the life you truly desire? Is it fear of success? Is it fear of failure? Is it the fear that you may not be good enough?

Fear is the one thing that stops people from engaging fully in their lives. Life is full of risks, and if someone lives in fear forever, are they truly living?

The truth is, the weight is a symptom of a deeper issue. For some people, it's an emotional issue, and for others, they've been on the cycle for so long, they don't know how to end the cycle to lose the weight permanently.

Once you've had bariatric surgery, it's time to deal with the emotional, psychological, and personal issues that arise post-surgery, so you can lose the weight for good. It's time to acknowledge the elephant in the room, which is not the weight, but the underlying issues that caused the weight gain to begin with.

Is this you?

Look back at each of the issues mentioned above, which ones resonate with you the most? Looking at your own life, which of these represents where you were or where you are?

Extreme obesity doesn't just happen overnight. It's something that happens over many years. We're going to delve deeper into your mindset and begin to shift your mindset to create a lifetime of success ahead of you after weight loss surgery (WLS).

You may have already begun, now it's time to really begin.

Building Awareness is the First Step

Where do we go from here?

Building awareness of your thoughts, feelings, and behaviors is the first step. This is where change begins.

You cannot change what you don't know. And, you don't know what you don't know. So, start reflecting on the last few years. What do you notice?

What does your life look like?

As you look at where you are, where you've been, and where you want to go in your own journey, take a deep look at your patterns of behavior.

What foods are your triggers?

What emotional states do you struggle with the most?

When do you crave foods that are not nutritionally sound?

Do you have a habit of sabotaging yourself when it comes to food or food triggers?

Asking yourself these questions, and writing down your answers in a personal journal, will help you recognize what you may not have seen all along, or what you subconsciously wanted to avoid.

I completely understand that while I'm over here preaching "awareness," you may be completely comfortable being oblivious. This is because once you are aware of something, you know you must change it and do something differently. For most people that's the hardest part of this process.

Wait … you mean I must change?

For a lot of people, living on autopilot is how they get through the day. Autopilot is just like it sounds. You wake up, eat breakfast, get ready for work, take the kids, go to work, have lunch, finish work, pick the kids up, get home, eat dinner, sit on the couch, get ready for bed, and repeat.

This day to day may sound completely boring, but when you take a good look at your life, how is it any different?

What is it that you want to see different for your life?

What would you like to gain in your life through all the weight that you lose?

That's why I'm using this book as a forum to share the strategies, techniques, and tools to help you be your most successful self, following weight loss surgery.

Coming from someone who is both a patient and a professional in the field, I offer two viewpoints: the one of the person who has been in your shoes and struggled with food and weight forever, yet overcome emotional eating, and the professional who has the strategies and tools to help you reach your next level.

I offer advice, info, and feedback. I also give you the unique point of view of "I've been there," and share the bird's-eye view of what I went through. While I honor that my journey may not be your journey, I hope that even though we are all different, I can share something that will help you through your journey.

I'm not saying my way will be your way; however, I'll share both my point of view and a general "here's what may likely happen," to help you with things to watch out for as you move along your own path. I offer suggestions for growth, I'll ask that you evaluate your feelings, and build on the awareness of your own experience to get the most out of this book.

Within my own practice, I like to offer my clients suggestions to "try on" – as some things will work, while some won't. You may have some strategies in this book work awesome for you while others are not your cup of tea. This is not designed to be a one size fits all, but a comprehensive guide to help you act within your own life, to be persistent with your process of lifestyle change.

It may not come easy, but I promise you that when you stick with it, the results are COMPLETELY worth it!

I hope this book serves you, your health, and your entire life. This book is not just about "how to lose weight and keep it off" or just about mindset …

This book is about setting you up for lifelong success following bariatric surgery, by helping you shift your mindset in the long term. I will encourage you to work on your habits and patterns every day, so you can achieve your own version of happiness.

Life after bariatric surgery is about living life fully and not going back to who or where you once were. It's about rebirth and creating the person you want to become through weight loss surgery.

You wanted this change for a reason, and it's important to remember it as you move through the chapters.

Chapter 2
Your New Bariatric Lifestyle & Your New Mindset
Changing Your Habits & Creating Lifestyle Change

"If you do what you've always done, you'll get what you've always gotten." – Tony Robbins

Prior to bariatric surgery, it's likely you did everything within your power to lose the weight. You've done all the diets, you've tried the pills, and you've probably eaten plastic food.

Yuck!

The old mantra of calories in, calories out is tried and true. You've got to eat less and exercise more. It's also likely that you've had a bazillion gym memberships, had a personal trainer at least once (if you could afford it), or own a series of fitness videos – now collecting dust in your home.

Whether you love or hate exercise, it's been a part of what you've been told to do over the years. As a former gym rat myself, I know the inside of the gym well.

In fact, I used to work in one. While in college, I was the front desk girl of a local gym. You know, the one who checks you in and out. I applied for the job since I spent a lot of time at the gym and figured … why not? I could do my homework while checking people in – oh, and don't forget the discounted membership! It sounded like a dream. I was told by an insider, that the owner did not think that I would be a good fit for the position, due to my weight.

He told the manager at the gym, "Fat people are generally lazy," but told her it was ultimately her choice. She gave me a shot, which I was grateful for. However, she gave me a heads-up by telling me this piece of information – mainly because she didn't want me to make her look bad.

I wasn't lazy; in fact, I was one of the best front desk people he ever had. I typically worked weekends at the gym due to a morning job I had during the week while also attending school in the evenings. It was about three years after my initial hire date that the owner personally approached me and recounted his hesitation to hire me. He went on to tell me that he was glad his manager made the decision to hire me because, using his words, "You are really awesome!"

I tell this story because being fat in this country is something we can be, and typically are, discriminated against for. There are stereotypes that linger, and judgments people make on your behalf – just based on your physical appearance. Knowing what I did at that time of my hire, I knew I had to work extra hard and show management and the owner that I wasn't lazy, and was in fact "worthy" of the job, despite my appearance.

This idea of "worthiness" will come up several times throughout this book, as it's one of the core issues many obese individuals deal with daily. Self-worth is a core belief and is the sense of one's own value or worth as a person, our self-esteem or self-respect.

If you don't have self-respect, or if you don't value yourself as a person, you tend to give things away for free. You find yourself doing things you have no business doing, and you do things that allow others to walk all over you. This has a lot to do with obesity, as I strongly believe, and clinical research indicates, that self-esteem and obesity are correlated (Klaczynski, Goold, & Mudry, 2004).

While self-esteem and obesity may impact one's self-belief or worth, they are all part of the cycle. Other parts of the cycle are emotional triggers and behaviors on autopilot.

Einstein said that the definition of insanity is "doing the same thing over and over and expecting different results."

This is no different with obesity. Knowing the cycle firsthand, I truly believed I was going crazy. I was at a loss for what to do next because nothing seemed to work.

Either I worked very, very hard to see little results, or I stopped attempting to change. I would experience extreme weight gain. It's important to note that there are biological factors and physiological factors at play, and I had no idea these factors existed until speaking with a bariatric surgeon.

I had no idea about hunger hormones (ghrelin and leptin) that lived in my stomach and sent messages to my brain that "Hey, we still have space down here!" I found this particularly interesting as I started conducting psychological/behavioral obesity research in bariatrics.

One study found while comparing nonobese populations to morbidly obese populations, that no observed differences in hunger were noted. However, it was observed that sleeve gastrectomy patients were less hungry and more satiated than the other groups (Mans, Serra-Prat, Palomera, Sunol, and Clave, 2015).

This same study also concluded that sleeve gastrectomy seemed to be associated with profound changes in gastrointestinal physiology, which contributes to reducing hunger and increasing sensations of satiation (Mans, Serra-Prat, Palomera, Sunol, and Clave, 2015).

This is a huge discovery, yet I must point out individuals cannot rely on the surgery alone, to cure their obesity problem. While both vertical sleeve gastrectomy and the RNY / gastric bypass procedures are shown to significantly reduce hunger and food intake due to the creation of a small pouch, it must be said that eating behaviors are largely responsible for weight regain.

Quite a few studies show that there are behavioral predictors of regain after bariatric surgery (Odom, et al., 2009). These behavioral predictors are a lack of self-monitoring (self-awareness), increased food urges, decreased well-being, and an increase in the use of alcohol/drugs or over-addictive behaviors (Odom, et al., 2009).

This means you don't know what you don't know.

If you are not recording your food, monitoring eating behaviors, and/or you have no clue what you are eating or drinking, over time you're likely headed toward regain. The research suggests that without continuous self-monitoring, and practiced self-awareness, individuals are not able to restrict themselves due to a lack of awareness of their behaviors.

The truth is, you cannot change what you're not aware of or do not know. As the saying goes, "If it's not broken, don't fix it." When someone is going through life unaware of their daily decisions, daily habits, then how could they possibly have the awareness to know they need to make a change?

Clearly, if over time, someone cannot fit into their jeans, this might give them a clue. But, why wait?

Get started on practicing your awareness early before it's too late. This is the first step in getting an inside view of your own mindset. Some of my clients are resistant to tracking their foods because they say, "I don't want to put myself under a microscope." This may be because they are used to being scrutinized by the food police in their home, or by a health-care provider. Regardless, to be most successful, you MUST track eating behaviors and caloric intake.

When my clients are resistant to this mindset, we work on awareness in our sessions, because they must learn that this process is for them and them alone. The process of tracking puts them in charge and is different from BEFORE surgery when they may have been judged for their eating.

Now, it's more about their success and if they are eating off track, it's something they need to be aware of so that we can get to the root of the issue.

Some of my clients eat off track, struggle with emotional eating issues, and turn to food as a coping mechanism. To help them discover the root of the issue, or issues, they need to recognize it's happening.

Avoidance is easy and comfortable; however, it doesn't help you or nurture growth. The numerous trips through the drive-through will not help you keep the weight off, so why make them? This behavior illustrates a deeper emotional attachment to food that needs to be addressed for the individual to be successful.

After bariatric surgery, you're given a strict diet to adhere to and follow. In the days and weeks following surgery, you'll transition from a liquid diet to soft foods, to semi-soft foods, and then a regular diet of hearty veggies and meats. In the initial phases, the diet restrictions are essential to get enough nutrients for the body to lose weight quickly, while going through the healing process from the surgery itself.

Bariatric Surgery and Nutrition

"Your stomach is not a wastebasket." – Author unknown

Following my vertical sleeve gastrectomy, I became a bit of a food snob. I decided that I would not put crap in my body anymore because my body deserved better. I avoid foods that are largely processed and try to stay with fresh proteins, fruits, and veggies. I stay away from fast food, and while I still like a good burger from time to time, it's not a regular on my menu.

When I do decide it's burger time, I avoid the bun and go for meat that is lower in saturated fat. By and large, I avoid simple carbs (stick with veggies!), and even when I visit my in-laws and my mother-in-law makes couscous, I eat very little of it. It's just not in my plan, so I focus on the protein first, just like the surgeon recommended, which has helped me stay on track.

The nutritional component is essential, because after bariatric surgery your body responds to food differently. One time I ate fast food in a pinch after totally forgetting to eat for several hours … I immediately regretted it.

I subsequently wrote a note in my food diary that day and highlighted it so that I'd remember how I felt. It was the most awful and disgusting feeling. My body felt heavy and lethargic. It was as though I was weighed down mentally and physically by cement bricks.

My body sent me this signal within 30 minutes, and in all my pre-surgery fast food experiences, I'd never ever felt this awful. Recording this helped me stay on track, so there are no repeats of the same behavior again.

My suggestion to you:

Avoid the crap!

If you do eat something and have a bad experience, write it down somewhere, or record it, so that you can avoid the behavior a second time. This is about progress, not perfection!

When you have bariatric surgery, you are essentially being placed into a state of nutritional deficit, and your body thinks it is starving because of a reduction of food intake. Therefore, it's essential you get the best nutrition possible, so your body will be running at optimal performance while losing weight.

This is another reason why fast food is not a good choice. The nutrition is low while the calories are high. The fat content is extremely high and can lead to dumping or the feeling I shared above. Ick! You may think you're getting the most bang for your buck in terms of cost, but you're not.

When you look at it from a nutritional perspective, you're feeding your body crap. This can lead to illness in the long term. Especially when digestive issues come up, sleep issues arise, and there's an increased likelihood that you'll return to obesity. These factors lead to other issues such as high blood pressure, diabetes, and/or joint issues, just to mention a few.

So, feeding your body foods high in nutrition, protein, vegetables, and fruits, for example, truly helps you to function at a maximum capacity, which in turn helps you live a better more fulfilling life.

If you're still hell-bent on drinking soda and eating foods high in carbohydrates or fat, and low in nutrition, please note that you will not be as successful as you could be, and you'll likely experience weight regain.

Since food can be an emotional issue, it's important that you get support from a professional, if you find you just can't kick these habits on your own. There are many professionals who help people with emotional eating change their habits, and for those with severe issues, food addiction. Also, keeping in touch with your surgeon or bariatrician's office would be important for additional support as well.

Most surgeons agree that soda is a bad idea for all bariatric patients, as the added sugar can impact blood sugar, and is generally a no-no. If you think you are exempt, speak with your doctor before buying the next 12 pack or 2-liter bottle. Many of the resources out there discuss the issues with carbonation and caffeine (in high doses). Therefore, it could impact your pouch negatively.

There is a reason you are here. If you're resistant to taking the required steps, or believe you have a medical reason for eating differently than what most surgeons recommend, talk with your doctor and discuss your situation for further clarification.

There are a ton of resources online that tell you how much protein you should eat, how much water you should drink, and how much exercise you need.

I'm going to share some of the basics, and then move on to the nitty-gritty details, which is your mindset. You'll find that I incorporate mindset into each point as well, because changing how you see things will help you change your actions, ultimately achieving the results you desire.

Protein

Protein and amino acids are the building blocks to muscle. The more muscle you have, the easier it is to burn fat. Additionally, when you have protein first, you feel full faster, giving your muscles what they need, avoiding muscle mass loss.

Every bariatric patient should be getting between 80–120 grams of protein per day. My surgeon's office recommended 100–120 grams of protein per day, while others may recommend 60–90 grams. Choosing protein-dense foods such as beef, pork, chicken, fish, tofu, or protein shakes, are important for your nutritional needs.

Please note, from my experience, beef is harder to digest. I could not eat beef for six months post-surgery. My body wouldn't let me. When I first ate beef following surgery (about 3 months out), I would have physical pains in my stomach. So, I listened to my body and stopped eating it.

You may be fine as this differs from person to person. Be sure to check with your physician or surgeon, on their recommendations when to reincorporate beef or beef products back into your diet following surgery.

Overall, protein is first and foremost the best choice in retaining muscle mass following surgery. Protein also helps you stay full longer and helps you lose more weight.

Vegetables

This is the food few people talk about in the WLS community, and is typically not the top five, in terms of requirements. Non-starchy vegetables are important for your health and well-being.

After surgery, the second most important food you should be eating after protein is vegetables. Low-glycemic vegetables like leafy greens (kale, spinach, etc.), veggies like broccoli, Brussel sprouts, cauliflower, and eggplant, are healthy choices. This is because they're high in fiber, a necessary component to your body's health.

You may not like vegetables; however, this is one of the ways your body gets the necessary nutrition. While supplements are great, vegetables contain the most natural form of vitamins. Your body can process these more efficiently. Eating vegetables is important, so finding creative and easy ways to prepare veggies will be in your best interest.

One of the quickest, and easiest, ways I found to get in the vegetables is by making a veggie and fruit smoothie with protein powder. Some of my clients have shared they don't like the taste of kale or spinach; however, throwing in half a banana, or some vanilla protein powder, can mask the taste while gaining the nutritional benefits.

Liquids

~ Water

Water is essential for the body. It's recommended you get at least 64 oz. per day, which is the equivalent of eight 8-oz. glasses. You can break this up in your day, by drinking a 4 oz. glass every 1/2 hour for 8 hours. You can set a timer as a reminder to make it easy.

Be sure to drink at least 30 minutes prior to eating and wait at least 30 minutes after eating to drink again. Eating and drinking together after bariatric surgery is not recommended. This is to ensure you get enough food to satiate. Additionally, no drinking is allowed while eating, to ensure fluids do not flush out the foods faster, causing you to overeat.

Getting your required water intake is important to manage hunger. Often when hunger strikes, it is masked as thirst. Therefore, drinking the recommended amount of water daily will help you stave off hunger pangs, keeping you hydrated. Bariatric patients tend to get dehydrated more easily than non-bariatric patients, so getting water in regularly throughout your day is essential.

~ Coffee/caffeine

The general rule is to wait at least 90 days post-op to ingest or consume caffeine, or to ask your surgeon. Some studies have shown there are issues with caffeine and nutrient absorption while others state that it's fine and doesn't inhibit hydration. It's best to check with your surgeon to confirm. Additionally, it's important to note that many caffeinated beverages are typically high caloric beverages that contain corn syrup or are high in sugar. Double-check with your dietitian or surgeon before resuming caffeine intake.

~ Alcohol and other substances

While there is a great debate regarding alcohol intake and bariatric patients, I recommend staying on the cautious side. The recommendation is to wait at least 3–6 months post-op before alcohol consumption. Alcohol is not a nutrient, it's a choice if you drink alcohol socially.

Personally, I don't recommend drinking following surgery. In my experience, and in speaking with some of my clients regarding their experience, when drinking, the alcohol hits you harder and faster. One drink as a post-op can feel like many. It's important to be especially cautious, because of the blood alcohol levels that show up in your bloodstream.

Your body will process the alcohol differently, and this could impact your ability to drive or operate heavy machinery. If you do plan on drinking after bariatric surgery, be sure that you have your first drink at home, so you're not put into a precarious situation or cause yourself legal trouble.

Within the bariatric community, there are some individuals who are subject to replacement behaviors or addiction transference. This means that instead of eating food, individuals may act out in other ways, such as using alcohol, drugs, sex/porn, shopping, or other harmful or addictive behavior.

If you believe you may have an addiction to alcohol, or any other substance/behavior, or if you believe you are transferring your pre-op eating behaviors to another area of your life that is creating problems for you, it is highly recommended that you reach out to a professional who can help you work on these issues.

Supplements

I'll start off by saying that I am not a physician, and the information I am presenting here is as a patient who has done extensive research. It is very important that you get the proper nutritional supplementation following bariatric surgery.

The type of nutritional support you need depends on the type of surgery you had. Bariatric surgery can put you in a physical state of nutritional deficiency. Therefore, it's important you have adequate supplemental nutrition support, in the form of vitamins and supplements geared toward bariatric patients.

Taking the same old vitamins as you did before surgery will not do as your body will have different needs. It's strongly suggested that you take specially formulated bariatric vitamins, to help your body get the nutrients it needs.

Avoid Slider Foods & Grazing

Slider foods are foods that are typically "snack" foods, that compress down when chewing and allow you to eat more. This increases your caloric intake without much awareness.

Examples of some of these foods are potato/tortilla chips, popcorn, crackers, and other snack type foods. These foods lead to grazing.

Grazing, or eating between meals, is a big no-no for bariatric post-op patients, as it leads to regain quickly. It's largely a function of emotional or mindless eating. The behavior is typically reminiscent of the days when you may have been sitting on the couch munching. Avoid slider foods … and avoid grazing.

In upcoming chapters, we'll discuss how to deal with head hunger, emotional eating, and food triggers.

Other Basic Elements for Your Weight Loss Success

~ Sleep

Getting adequate sleep is essential for anyone's weight loss plan. If you're struggling to get your Zs, there may be something else going on, and you may want to check in with your doctor.

The Mayo Clinic recommends between 7 to 9 hours of sleep per night for adults. Adequate sleep helps your body to repair itself. Studies have shown that sleep deprivation is linked to weight gain; therefore, getting the necessary amount of restful sleep is essential for individuals looking to lose or maintain their weight (Hensrud, 2015).

~ Checking in with your doctor (surgeon, bariatrician, PCP)

Talking to your doctors and dietitians on staff will provide you with added support if you are unsure or have questions. If you have any doubts about vitamin supplements, your food intake, water intake, or what to eat / not eat, call your surgeon's office, physician's office, or bariatrician's office. Your doctor's office is a great resource, with a wealth of information.

In successive chapters, we'll talk about creating a plan that includes techniques to incorporate these recommendations into your diet and lifestyle. Getting the protein, water, vegetables, nutrients, and supplements are essential for your dietary needs.

Furthermore, the exercise component is equally important for strengthening your body, building muscle, and creating lean body mass so your body can efficiently burn fat.

The Therapeutic Component

Sometimes talking things out with friends or dropping into a support group is simply not enough. Each person is different, so determining if a therapeutic approach is right for you would be key.

After I had surgery, I spoke with a therapist that practiced within my bariatric surgical center, a few times. However, when I realized I needed deeper, more intense sessions, I decided to work with someone who could see me more often.

Therapists, counselors, and even psychologists can be a wealth of knowledge, support, and accountability for individuals struggling to make changes after surgery. As you may have come to realize, there is more than the eating and behavioral changes needed to be successful.

There are issues with relationships, family, friends, career, and so on. Having someone who is unbiased, and whose entire focus is on you, can be helpful for you. Seeing things from another perspective, that you may not have otherwise seen, heard, or been privy to, without that relationship, can be beneficial.

It's also important to know that therapists/counselors are different from coaches. Not every therapist/counselor or psychologist is a coach. Sometimes it's a benefit to have both because therapists/counselors empathize, helping you see things differently, and help you go back to the past, to help you overcome issues haunting you. They can help you move past trauma.

Coaches, however, do better at holding you accountable, calling you out on your excuses, and help you set goals that are achievable. Counseling is very past/present-oriented, whereas coaching is very present/future-oriented.

The therapy/counseling industry is regulated by state licenses, and each therapist/counselor or psychologist must obtain a minimum number of years in school.

The field of coaching is not regulated like that, causing many coaches to pop up out of nowhere. Coaching can be very beneficial; however, it's important if you decide to hire a coach, that the person you work with is trained in bariatrics and not just someone who had surgery and believes they are an expert.

Look at their credentials to see if they've attended a board-certified coaching program, or a coaching program that requires them to practice a specific number of hours. If your coach has letters behind his/her name, ask them what they mean, and ask them where they received their training. This will help determine if they are skilled trained professionals and not someone who's hung up their shingle indiscriminately.

Exercise

The key to your success is exercising consistently and starting the program early. By early I mean, by the time you've hit the 90-day point following surgery. Right after surgery, your body is in shock, and while getting your body in motion, high-level cardio or weight lifting is not recommended.

It's highly recommended by surgeons and bariatricians that you wait at least 60–90 days before starting an exercise program, so your body has time to heal, and you've adjusted to the reduction in calories.

The easiest way to start exercise post-surgery is to make sure that you are exercising and getting yourself in the mindset before surgery – even by starting a simple workout routine prior to surgery.

By being proactive you will be toned, happy (think endorphins), and stronger. Another important thing to note is when you're going through the process of bariatric surgery, exercise and your eating plan are going to be a part of a new life.

You want to make sure that you are starting a new and consistent pattern of exercise, even in the smallest of doses in the beginning. The key here is to make sure that you can get into a pattern of exercise, even just 5–10 minutes per day prior to the 90-day mark is sufficient.

This will give you the consistency of building a new habit. One thing that's important to realize is exercise brings improved quality of life. If you're focusing on losing weight, and on feeling better, doing something as simple as walking can ensure you're going to boost your mood. You're going to have an easier transition and ensure that you keep the weight off.

There are many people who think that they are going to be able to lose weight and keep it off without exercise. This is definitely something that is important because exercise is the way to make sure that the weight stays off. There are many people who think that they are going to find a way to outsmart biology and this is not the case. Exercise is a part of life if you want to make sure that you are going to keep the weight off. What that also means is that it is very important to ensure that you are going to have access to activities that you are going to enjoy.

~ Exercise and self-talk

When it comes to thinking about exercise, the key to success is making sure you're enjoying the activities. Many people start out disliking exercise because of the pain or discomfort from the excess weight they're carrying around.

Others have shared with me, they've always disliked exercise. To be successful, exercise must be part of the program. It's something that's going to be a part of your life, and therefore it's important you find something you'll enjoy.

Therefore, starting small as discussed above, is so essential. No one is running a 5K right after surgery. While many WLS patients do end up running marathons and 5K races, they do so after a process of conditioning their body over time. You don't have to be a runner or a 5K champion to have a routine.

You only need yourself and the habit of exercise. Creating a habit out of exercise will help you because when you have days that are a struggle, you'll know exactly how to overcome the excuses.

There are many people who may exercise for a while and then they go back to their old situations and habits. It's very important to ensure that you focus on how to keep yourself motivated. You need to see when you're making excuses, that's what's happening, and you need to bust through the excuses right away, allowing you to move forward, not backward.

If you allow yourself to take time off from your routine, you will find yourself in the situation of excuses. When someone makes the mistake of taking too many days off, it's very easy to fall back into old patterns, and before you know it you have lost the momentum of your success.

Many people will drift away from their routine and struggle with success in other areas as well. Additionally, they will lose the drive they had, leading them to make other poor choices. One thing inevitably leads to another.

This the mantra of many people pre-surgery. Many people lose their routine and when that happens, they'll say the "diet" never worked … even though what happened was they returned to their old habits.

The difference now is that this is not a diet …

This is a lifestyle change.

Inside your head, there is resistance.

Emotional resistance is that little voice inside your head that says, "I don't want to."

When this voice is loud, typically nothing gets done. This lets you know you are resistant. There can be many reasons you don't like exercise, you don't want to exercise, or you just don't feel like it.

Motivation is built over time, it's not something that comes and sits on your shoulder like people believe. Many people wait to do something, waiting for the motivation to arrive. When people tell me this, I assure them that they could be waiting forever.

It's like creativity or inspiration, if you wait for it, life may pass you by. Therefore, acting, in fact, is one of the best ways to become motivated. You will get an emotional boost from the activity itself.

It shows that you, in fact, CAN DO, whatever it is that you put your mind to. By taking action, you bust through the emotional barriers of "I just can't" because in fact, you can, and you just did. In turn, you'll have proof that you can do it again.

Thus, mindset is powerful.

As Henry Ford famously stated, "Whether you think you can, or you think you can't, you are right!"

Self-belief is integral to your new bariatric mindset. Your belief systems are being overhauled. The old ways of doing things are no longer going to serve you. The old patterns of thinking will not get you where you want to go.

There's another saying I love dearly that sums this up, "What got you here, won't get you there!" In essence, your old behaviors will not lead you to the success you desire; you must do something differently.

This is so true because eating fast food and sitting on your couch will not help you lose weight. Likewise, the excuses, rationalizations, and permissions to continue the cycle of poor habits will not get you to where you want to be.

This is where our mindset work begins!

Consciously, I know you know all of what I'm saying. Your subconscious mind, however, is a bit trickier.
Your subconscious mind houses your belief systems, which are hidden below the surface. So, while you know something on a conscious level, you might still not believe it at a subconscious level.

Busting Up Excuses

Many times, we find ourselves in the middle of excuses ... here is what we can do to overcome those excuses.

Remember your health is number one.

Tell yourself that you need to remember your health is improving day by day with exercise, and it's beneficial to get your body in motion, even by starting small. Make a list of how you would benefit by putting your health first. By changing how you think about health, fitness, and your post-operative journey, you will likely gain a lot of new insights. Many tend to focus on the discomfort or the time it will take. Sure, if you focus on that, then yes, it will be hard to get off the couch. However, if you focus on how good you will feel and look, and create ways to integrate healthy living into your current lifestyle, you will find it to be easier than you think.

Focus on Your Ideal Self.

Make sure you have an image of what you want to look like and that you're looking at it on a regular basis. This will help you remind yourself why you are working out. Also, get into the feelings of how good you will feel as your ideal self. By getting into the emotions of the excitement of your ideal self, this can also help you shift your thinking to get moving.

We are all short on energy these days. Remember that working out will help you have more of it and that you will have it increase over the days to come. Shift your thinking to who you want to be, and how movement will help you get there.

Exercise and youth!

If you are looking to be healthier, and you want to make sure you're being as young as possible, know you are going to be able to take care of yourself by using exercise to turn back the hands of time. Exercise can help you feel and look younger. Exercise helps skin elasticity and there are some studies which show it boosts collagen production. Therefore, exercise can help you to look and feel younger despite the effort it takes.

All too often we may make excuses to exercise, but it is important to remember what it is you are doing. Meaning, you are hurting yourself when you know that exercise is the long-term key to your success. Imagine putting off something like going to the doctor, or holding off on doing something you do every day … exercise is in this same classification even if it doesn't seem like it in the moment.

Starting Your Exercise Program

When you start a new program, you need to know it is going to take you approximately six months to a year to create a pattern. Most people believe it takes 28–30 days to create a habit; however, when you're rewiring your brain from a pattern of not exercising to a pattern of exercising, it takes a lot more time to get you moving forward. Consequently, commitment to exercise and your weight loss success program is key!

In addition to that, you need to know that there are huge benefits to starting the routine. In the beginning you may not look forward to exercising, but you will see an increase in energy once you get moving.

Exercise is great for the heart, it is great for the mind, your mood, and it will ensure new levels of control over your situation. When you are starting a new program, it's going to be hard getting used to ensuring you are putting yourself first, and that you are focusing on the way you're going to work with your situation.

You need to realize if you are having insurance pay for your surgery, you must look at the investment coming from the company, and know that you have a team who is there to support you in your venture. You have the nurses, the doctor, your pre-op psychologist, and many others who are there to help you with the process.

Your New Mindset After the Honeymoon is Over

Once you've landed the first steps of bariatrics and weight loss surgery with these post-surgical basics, it's time to dig deeper into what will really hold you back: your mindset.

The previously mentioned requirements will determine the difference in a successful surgical post-op and someone who experiences regain.

You might ask why would post-op patients not do the above requirements post-surgery?

The answer: mindset.

The right mindset is required for a long-term lifestyle change. Lifestyle change is the ultimate success tool; however, to master your new habits, you've got to get past the honeymoon phase.

Initially, you'll start off with liquids, then mushy foods, then soft foods, then you'll integrate more solid foods, as you work up to eating real foods again mentioned earlier in this chapter. As you may know from reading online and visiting your surgeon's office, this is a long process. I'm not sharing all the details about this here, because that is not the focus of this book.

The focus of this book is to help you with the psychological, emotional, behavioral, and strategic pieces long after the honeymoon phase is over, and once you've integrated real food back into your diet.

This will be called your NEW NORMAL.

The new normal is committing to the plan given to you by your surgeon's office, their dietician or nutritionist, and to implement this plan long after you've gone home from surgery following your recovery. This piece is largely behavioral in nature.

In the short term, you'll see the weight loss. However, as you get back to normal, the old habits can begin to creep in …

Unless you change your mindset.

You'll go to parties, you'll get back to long days at the office, and you might even forget to prep your food for the week. The result? You could be subject to making poor choices that are the quick and easy options.

Before you say, "Oh, no! That would never be me!"

Don't be so quick to judge in either direction. No one is on their good behavior 100% of the time, and none of us are perfect. There will be slips. There will be mishaps. This is life.

Let's get real with each other. I know, and you know, you will have cake in your mouth again at some point in your life. I'm not a fool and please do not fool yourself to think it won't happen. The difference in having cake in your mouth twice a year versus once a week depends on your mindset.

If you haven't shifted your mindset, you'll justify the poor choices and quick eats because you'll see it as a short-term solution. However, as this occurs repeatedly, you'll end up with the reemerging pattern of behavior eating junk once again. Only this time, you're eating less of it because your stomach is smaller.

The nutrition you need is not in the quick fixes or the short-term emergency options. The nutrition you need is built from the conscious decisions you make, not the autopilot decisions you make because of poor planning.

Everyone knows that phrase, "When you fail to plan, you plan to fail."

This is NOT what I want for you. Mindset must be addressed to help you shift your patterns of behavior and get a hold of the daily steps so that you can ensure your successful self, following surgery.

Equally, the notion of "I don't have time to plan" is simply an excuse because where there is a will, there is a way. Planning is an essential component of reaching your goals and we'll cover the majority of that in the next chapter.

Before you can plan, you must be conscious of your decisions. As I shared earlier, most people are on autopilot. Your mindset and intention for what you want need to be thought of and discussed.

Each decision that occurs, is either a product of your autopilot behaviors, or habits. Therefore, the goal throughout this book is to give you tips, techniques, and strategies to help change your habits. It will help you remove the autopilot thinking.

There will still be days that are a struggle.

Understandable. That's life.

However, when you create new habits that shift your behaviors you will start to see outstanding results. You'll see when struggles pop up because you have healthy habits in place, the resistance isn't so strong.

The mindset shift begins to occur.

Chapter Review and Exercises

1. What exercises do you enjoy?

2. What exercises can you do daily without equipment or spending money? (More on this in chapter 3)

3. What "aha" moments have you experienced regarding your current eating, lifestyle, or exercise behaviors?

4. What do you think you need to change?

Important Elements

❖ Keep your nutrition high

❖ Focus on protein first

❖ Drink your water

❖ Watch your carbs, sugar, and fat

❖ Get your sleep

Chapter 3

Creating a Plan and Setting Your Intentions for Long-Term Success

At 32 years old, at five feet four inches and at over 380 lb., Elizabeth sat in my office describing how she felt like a total failure. She shared how she set goals over and over each New Year's Eve, and how by February 10th, she was back into her old patterns, completely oblivious, confused, and disappointed.

"For the last 10 years, I feel like I'm in the same place, going nowhere, except each year, I lose less and gain more!"

The frustration in her voice told me she felt destroyed, and that she feared she might never achieve her weight loss goals. However, once we dissected how she'd been setting her goals, we both realized very quickly, that she'd been setting them all wrong.

She'd been setting herself up for failure from the start. It wasn't about working harder, and usually never is. It's about having a strategic plan in place to help you expect, anticipate, and overcome the obstacles that pop up along the way, so you can reach your goals, no matter what!

As a bariatric patient myself, I remember thinking to myself, "How am I going to lose 50, 100, 150 or even 200 lb.?"

By the time I'd reached my top weight, I think I'd just about given up, because what could I possibly do to make the change?

The weight would come off 5 lb. at a time. Then it would just stop, despite my best efforts of having a personal trainer, food portioned, and making food, eating, and dieting my entire world. This is where surgery came in to help me achieve success; however, it wasn't surgery alone. Along with the mindset shifts, I reached long-term weight loss success.

The reality is, for someone who has that much weight to lose, they will likely need bariatric surgery to help them gain the momentum needed to lose the weight for good. This has been the case for many of my clients, who have shared they've felt the same way.

Often, it's the mixture of behavioral and biological effects that prevent people from losing massive amounts of weight. Again, this is where weight loss surgery really helps the severely obese to lose the weight.

It's not surgery alone that allows long-term permanent weight loss. It's the mindset work and behavioral shifts / habit changes, that make the biggest difference once you've had surgery. I know in my own experience, the surgery has been amazing in helping me maintain control over my stomach while building control within myself.

See, as I stated earlier, the surgery is not a "fix-all "…

It's a tool and a guide that helps people regain control of themselves, their eating, and their lives.

Did you know that only about 20% of individuals who are able to lose weight without surgery, keep it off long term? (Wing & Phelan, 2005)

Even then, their total weight loss is only about 10% of their total body weight (Wing & Phelan, 2005). It's important to note that without bariatric surgery, many people return to their old behavior. They are working so incredibly hard to lose the weight, and with very little visible evidence of success either on the scale or in their clothes – they give up.

The path of weight loss is much different from weight maintenance. Therefore, it's easy to see why and how people regress back to their former selves. With bariatric surgery, however, people can still regress if they engage in a free-for-all, and not use the guidelines recommended by their surgeons, bariatrician, and/or dietitian/nutritionist.

Therefore, setting a long-term plan for success begins with a short-term plan that requires one to be more present, conscious, and aware of their behaviors, feelings, habits, and practices.

Creating a plan that fosters awareness is important so that you aren't standing in the middle of your life five years from now with a blank stare on your face asking, "What went wrong?" or "How did I get here?"

That's precisely why you are here, and this, my dear, is your wake-up call. Are you ready to take charge and live your best life after WLS?

Goal Setting Basics

For many bariatric patients, goals are not a foreign concept. It's likely you've worked on your weight loss goals long before you ever thought about surgery as an option.

It's likely you know what your goals are. Yet, you are probably cynical, since up until now, it's been hard to reach them. Following bariatric surgery, it gets easier because you see the amazing progress and you see it quickly. There are stalls in weight, which can freak people out.

"Am I stuck? Will I continue to lose? Is this a plateau? How long will I be here (at this weight)?"

The panic sets in.

First, calm down. If you are doing what needs to be done, your weight will continue to drop. As you lose the weight, your body is adjusting to a sharp decrease in food intake. You may want to discuss with your surgical team (bariatrician, dietician, etc.) regarding how many calories you are getting and whether you need to decrease or increase your caloric intake.

You may be shocked at this but sometimes the reason people are not losing weight is that they are simply not eating enough and the body has engaged in starvation mode so it is hanging on to every morsel in your body. Other times, you may need to reduce your calories to continue to experience weight loss. This is a very personal issue and stalls do happen.

We all experience them. Some people experience stalls that last two weeks and some people experience stalls that last six weeks. This is when it's important to reach out to your physician or dietitian to evaluate what you may or may not be doing to help you drop. This is why awareness is important. If you are eating off-plan and not aware, you're returning to autopilot behavior that may be causing you to gain the weight.

Another study found that when people were engaged in self-monitoring, they did a better job of losing weight and keeping the weight off (Odom, et al., 2009). Self-monitoring consists of keeping a food journal, tracking exercise and other progress, as well as tracking water intake, supplements, and emotions.

It's a good idea to grab a food journal to track your eating, on a day-to-day basis, so you are practicing the awareness of what you are eating. This helps you consciously process what you are about to put into your mouth or reflect on what you already ate on any given day. It's been shown that when you are more conscious of your choices, you make better ones.

It is important to be realistic about your goals, and it's essential that you discuss this with your surgeon as well. I also need to note here, for some individuals the BMI chart can be deceiving.

This does not mean you get a free pass to bypass the BMI chart; however, it's important to see where you fall and whether it's a factor in your actual body fat percentage overall. As someone who is five feet eleven inches tall, I know I'm never going to be 160 lb., and that is exactly what the chart shows I should be. I'm not saying that you should hide your head in the sand, or state you're "big-boned " if you're not.

The goal is for you to lose weight and to be healthy for your body's height. It's all about proportion. The goal here is NOT to get you down to a specific weight per se, but to get you to a weight that YOU are comfortable at, and at a weight and size in which you feel good living in your body. You, feeling comfortable in your own body, makes all the difference.

Let's look at your personal goals for the short term and long term, to help you gain an idea of where you want to be.

~ What are the realistic goals for your weight and height?

~ How much do you expect to lose overall?

~ What is your HEIGHT?

~ What was your HIGHEST weight?

~ What was your surgery weight?

~ What is your current weight?

~ What is your ideal ending goal weight?

~ What are your post-surgery (pounds lost) goals for:

Month 1:

What size do you want to be in?

How do you want to feel?

Month 3:

What size do you want to be in?

How do you want to feel?

Month 6:

What size do you want to be in?

How do you want to feel?

Month 9:

What size do you want to be in?

How do you want to feel?

Month 12:

What size do you want to be in?

How do you want to feel?

Month 18:

What size do you want to be in?

How do you want to feel?

Month 24:

What size do you want to be in?

How do you want to feel?

Month 30:

What size do you want to be in?

How do you want to feel?

Month 36:

What size do you want to be in?

How do you want to feel?

If you don't know what you want, how will you go after it?

Clarity is so important. Knowing what you want is step one. If you do not yet know what you will do once you lose the weight, start thinking about it now.

Clearly, the plan is to lose weight and to do all the things you have not had the opportunity to do as an obese individual. There's so much more life for you to live and many things that I know you want to do.

~ Do you have a desire to travel in Europe and walk through the ancient streets of Rome?

~ Do you want to walk/run a 5K?

~ Do you want to chase after your grandchildren and be able to pick them up at a moment's notice?

~ Or would you like to feel comfortable making love to your husband/wife?

~ What is it that means the most to you?

~ What are those things that you're excited to do now that you're losing the weight?

Get out a sheet of paper and list them out.

How to Set Goals Appropriately

While most people suggest you go for SMART goals (SPECIFIC, MEASURABLE, ACHIEVABLE, RELEVANT, & TIME BOUND), if the goals are too large, or too far out in terms of time, people get lost in trying to achieve them, become overwhelmed, bored, or completely lose motivation with the process. Setting SMART goals alone, for some, ends up being a bust.

It's not completely about setting SMART goals, but adding accountability and some steps along the way so that you can see progress. It's also about estimating and establishing short-term progress and taking chances as you move forward when the status quo becomes less than exciting.

For example, instead of setting a 100-lb. weight loss goal that could take you 7–12 months to achieve after WLS, set a 10-lb. weight loss goal within a specific frame of time, and build up the excitement to get to the next step.

Beginning with the end in mind, an old Stephen Covey habit, is a great way to get started; however, your goals may change over time, and that's OK (Covey, 1998). Let's say you start out with the desire that you'll be a triathlete by the time you get to your goal, when midway through your process you realize you absolutely hate running. Don't get down on yourself, just shift gears and change your plan so that you have a goal you are super excited about!

Don't give up, just change the goal!

Visualize the Outcome You Desire

Visualizations have been around for years. There is scientific evidence, showing people who utilize visualizations are more likely to achieve their goals. Visualizations are used to create a detailed mental image of the desired outcome using all your senses (Canfield, 2015).

In fact, sports psychologists use visualizations as part of their treatment protocol when helping their clients achieve the next level, or when they are helping them reach a breakthrough in training. There has been evidence to suggest that when runners visualize running their course, their muscles are firing in the same way they would be firing as if they were running the course.

Our minds are extremely powerful, so this is a great technique to use to our advantage. In fact, Olympic athletes use visualizations to program their subconscious minds toward achieving their goals.

The reason that visualization is so important is that it taps into your reticular activating system (RAS), which helps in reprogramming your subconscious mind. Your mind thinks in pictures, not words, and therefore by activating your RAS, your brain is picturing images just like you would in a movie.

When conducting visualizations, experts suggest that the more of your senses you use, the more real it makes it feel, and thus creates this reality in your actual life. What you visual in your mind, you can achieve in your life, because your subconscious mind is working out the details.

When you use all your senses – sight, sound, tastes, and smells – you multiply the effects of the visualization. When you add emotions, such as how you would feel in this situation, the body sensations that you feel would be akin to what it's like when you've achieved that outcome.

Think of a time from your childhood when you were happy, an event of sorts. Maybe it was that Christmas morning when you got a dog, or a new dollhouse. Or maybe it was the moment that you got the highest grade in the class, or your friends gathered around to cheer you on.

Whatever your memory, look back and remember how you felt. Visualize the memory and recall how you felt and recall what else you noticed in that moment as a sensory experience. What did you see? Was there a taste, smell, or sound to the memory?

Now, shift your attention to the future. Think of something that you'd like to take place but hasn't happened yet. Visualize yourself at your perfect weight and take a snapshot in your mind. Maybe it's when you are kayaking across a lake. Or maybe you are at a party with friends. Wherever you envision, take a snapshot of this moment and project your senses into this moment.

What are you wearing? Use details.

What are you feeling?

Are you happy, excited, or elated?

What sounds, smells, or tastes can you experience in this moment?

Get clear on your emotions and use your senses to get into the experience. The more you use your senses, the better sensory experience you have. The more focus you have on visualizing the moment, the more powerful your results will be. This helps you be more present and aware of that moment because you were in touch with the sensation of that visualized event.

In Jack Canfield's book *The Success Principles,* chapter 11 specifically, he discusses the reticular activating system and using the first 10 minutes of your day to produce a significant outcome over time (Canfield & Switzer, 2015). Visualizations are a powerful tool for getting your day started, and while it may seem like daydreaming, the scientific evidence that backs it up, proves it's is hardly fleeting.

I'll be adding a visualization exercise in chapter 6, so you can practice this even more!

Get Clear on Your "WHY" and Stay away from "Why?"

Your big WHY is the reason you are here. It's the whole reason you had weight loss surgery. There is something deeper within you that has caused you to say, "Enough is enough." Weight loss surgery is a huge lifestyle shift and to be successful, you need to be clear on your WHY.

Your WHY is not necessarily one thing, but the deeper reasons or reasoning that you called on something so drastic as bariatric surgery to help you lose weight.

For me, it was my son and husband. I had trouble walking and breathing when I walked. My foot and knee pain when I walked was excruciating. I had trouble carrying my infant son, fearing I might fall and hurt him and myself. There comes a time when the pain is greater to stay the same than it is to make a change. This time came when my husband told me that we needed to pursue weight loss surgery, not because of vanity, but because he feared for my life.

My WHY is my family and my life. As a weight loss surgery patient, I've regained my life and so much more. As an active individual, I can go anywhere and do anything. I fly regularly, feeling comfortable in a tiny single airline seat, and it's comfortable to walk miles without fearing that my feet or ankles might swell.

You may be tempted to focus on the other "Why" – and for clarity purposes, I'm writing them differently, so you know the difference. The other "Why" is your need to understand the reasons behind your eating behaviors. The truth is, knowing your "Why" is not necessarily going to change your eating behaviors. Although, sometimes they help you build the awareness enough to say "Oh, that's the reason, let's do something about it."

However, an overwhelming majority of individuals who want to know their "Why" don't really get out of the rut they are in. While awareness is important, the behavior you want to change also has triggers. The trigger prior to your behavior is the antecedent.

In behavioral psychology there is the:

(A) Antecedent

(B) Behavior

(C) Consequence

In the case of weight loss and weight gain, you have triggers to eat, which are antecedents. Then you have the consequence, which is either weight gain or weight loss. If you are triggered by anxiety (antecedent) and eat a tub of ice cream (behavior), you'll likely gain weight (consequence).

When we learn to respond instead of react, we can change the behavior when there is a trigger, and do something different. So, when you are triggered with anxiety (antecedent), and you practice the awareness to respond differently, then your behavior may be to go for a walk or call a friend.

You will automatically use another coping mechanism to soothe yourself, changing the trajectory of your result, allowing for the greater probability of weight loss and avoiding weight gain. This process takes time as this is also the reprogramming of your subconscious mind through mindset shifts.

Just like the old behavioral example of Pavlov's dog being trained to salivate when hearing the bell, we too can condition our subconscious mind to respond differently to food, food triggers, and alter our eating behaviors. This helps us change the way we look at food as well.

The old thinking that I modeled before bariatric surgery was to put foods into the "good" and "bad" categories. This also make some of those "bad" foods even more desirable. It made me want them more. At that time, I also did not realize the impact they had not my body. I ate purely for emotional satisfaction with little regard to how protein, fat, or carbs impacted my body. The desire and sensations for what I wanted came with urgency. It was a highly emotional process.

The first part of the learning came in learning how to heal the emotional urges with something other than food. Just because the urge was present did not dictate that I had to eat. Instead, I have gathered tools to help me surf the urges when they strike and deal with the emotional triggers separate from food. This process allowed me to build new neuropathways so that I did not return to food to cope with my feelings. Another lesson learned was practicing the art of slowing down in order to take a step back and reflect. This allowed me to change my perspective *of food* which has helped me to alter my relationship *with food*.

After surgery, I've processed looking at food with different eyes. I don't see food as bad or good, instead, I see it as pouch-worthy, or not pouch-worthy. I look at how the food will make me feel after I eat it. You can also ask yourself these questions too. Is this food nutritious and nourishing? Will it help fuel me throughout the rest of my day? Or will this food bring me down? Will it make me feel energetically heavy, dense, or like I need a nap? This is a helpful determining factor in deciding what to eat, especially after surgery.

As we have limited space after WLS, I look for foods that are both tasty and nutritious, as I've shared previously. Once you start on this process too, as many of my clients have, it becomes fun to see what you can eat today that fills you up and tastes good.

I like to think of this as, what you "GET" to eat instead of what you "HAVE" to eat. This shifts the whole paradigm of thinking and creates a mindset shift within your brain that builds a positive relationship with food and eating behaviors.

Past/Future Self – Creating a Plan

"If you do what you've always done, you'll get what you've always gotten." – Tony Robbins

You had bariatric surgery to create change in your life. If you wanted to stay heavy forever, you would not have had the surgery.

I can completely relate because when I began my bariatric/WLS journey, I was so done with being obese. I thought that once I lost the weight, all my problems would disappear. And, of course, they didn't.

The weight was just a symptom of my overarching problem.

Me. My behaviors. My habits. My fears.

The problem was my emotions, and how I coped with them.

Dealing with them, however, was something totally different. I'm talking about this here because you'll need a plan. My clients have shared similar feelings, which is why I've created this book.

My goal is to reach more people, to share that you are not alone, and you can create a new reality by recognizing the mindset shifts that lead you to success. You'll reach the messy middle, feel stuck, and confused about your next steps.

This is where your plan comes in. It's your resource, your tool, and your friend. Planning is the bariatric person's best-kept secret, because it helps you stay on track while also enjoying the food you eat.

In chapter 2, I talked about the fundamentals of bariatric/WLS in terms of what you'll need to be successful. There are two parts, your mindset, and your tools (protein, water, exercise, supplements, and support).

Your mindset is important for your success. How you begin to craft your mindset, will be through creating a strategic success plan for yourself. Even as someone who has struggled with planning for years, I recognized that part of my failure to keep weight off was because I planned poorly and would end up with last resort eating, usually at a drive-through.

I'll say it again, "When you fail to plan, you plan to fail."

I'm here to encourage you to create a plan so that you can be successful in the long term. Now that I'm a planner, and encourage my clients to plan, they are wildly successful. They are amazed at how it doesn't take that much time at all.

Usually, the initial resistance I get from new clients, is they spend so much time planning. I believe that you can have things that are quick and easy while also being successful, it's just a matter of strategy. This process is not about working harder, but instead working smarter. I'm all about keeping things super simple for your success.

This plan begins with your list of protein-rich foods from which you can access at any time.

Grab my go-to easy protein sources on my blog at Bariatric Mindset or see appendix A.

Make sure you add your own suggestions to the list so that you will have a complete list of quick/easy and healthy foods you can grab at a moment's notice.

Also, make a list of the meals you and your family like the most. Use this as your guide. Also, look on Pinterest for bariatric-friendly ways to make each one. Most recipes have bari-friendly versions.

For example, instead of chicken fried rice, you may find a bariatric-friendly version that is cauliflower fried rice with chicken. Instead of lasagna, you can find bariatric lasagna sans noodles, or with zucchini noodles (also known as zoodles). This is about creativity and having fun with your food, so you can lose weight and enjoy the process.

Again, this is not about deprivation or trying harder – this process is about lifestyle change and using what you like and modifying them for your new bariatric lifestyle.

Meal Planning

Each week I sit down on Saturday and create my meal plan for the week. On Sunday I go shopping and prepare my food for the week. I can say that this has helped me most with planning and preparing food for the week.

Are there weeks when this doesn't happen? Yes.

However, those are the weeks that I see I am most tempted and struggle the most. The mindset piece is very real, and when life is not planned, things can go haywire.

No one is perfect, present company included! I don't claim to be perfect, but I do claim to have a system that works when I work it!

Therefore, it's important to plan out your meals for the week.

And, I know what you may say as an objection, "But, I don't know what I'll want to eat on Thursday, or I can't eat the same thing all week."

I have an answer to all of this. Variety!

It's important to plan, and account for things like food boredom, variety, nights that you may work late, your child's swim lessons, ballet night, or if you are traveling.

These things can be accounted for, and yes, you can plan for them. Unfortunately, there will be situations you cannot plan for. When those situations arise, you'll still be prepared because you'll have such a good system going, you'll be encouraged to stay on track.

Steps for success:

Step 1: Get out a sheet of paper and mark down the days of the week.

Step 2: Create a table, write out columns or breakfast, lunch, and dinner and write out rows for days of the week

Step 3: Write in your meal planning ideas for each meal

Step 4: Create a grocery list based on your weekly meal plan

Step 5: Take action – go to the grocery store and buy the foods to make your meal plan for the week

Breakfast and lunch will likely be on your own, while dinner will most likely be a family meal, so choose meals that are bari-friendly and family-friendly.

You can do both!

Or you can grab your very own *Bariatric Mindset Success Accountability Workbook* available for purchase through my Author Page at Amazon. All you'll need to do is fill in the blanks with your meal plan.

Take your list of bari-friendly dinners and place them throughout the week. It's good to have three dinners planned throughout the week with two leftover nights so you're not cooking every night.

Or, you can preplan your meals on a Sunday, so you're cooking less during the week and more on a single day. This process varies depending on your schedule and what works for you. You can cook weekly or a few times a week. You may try it a few different ways to see what works best for you, your family, and your schedule.

Rely on Discipline over Willpower

Most often when you've given yourself permission to go off track for too long, it's hard to get back on track. However, when you prepare and plan for all sorts of situations, you're consistently prepared and encouraged to eat healthy even when there is a day when plans go out the window.

It's better to be disciplined than to depend on willpower.

Willpower tends to lose every time; however, when you are disciplined, you'll eat well even when you slip. It will be far easier to catch yourself and put yourself back on track when slips happen. Discipline requires practice, and it's the practice over time for which you gain more control.

This process is about being more conscious of your day-to-day activities rather than leaving things to chance. When things are left to chance, we both know there is the possibility for all hell to break loose, and you could be headed to a drive-through. To avoid that, planning will help you stay disciplined and on track to avoid pitfalls, or slipping into old habits.

Relying on willpower alone is a dangerous and slippery slope because the mind was previously programmed to go for what you desire in that moment, which may not always be the healthiest choice. Once you plan and have disciplined yourself to think ahead about the food and its health benefits, you can enjoy a tasty and healthy meal without guilt or fear.

Use a meal planner to plan your meals ahead. This will help you to feel more in control and lead you to practice the planning process. When you think ahead about the food, you'll feel more in charge to make better choices in the long run.

Exercise Planning

Just like meal planning, you've got to plan to exercise. Your health is a priority and when you utilize excuses like "I don't have time," this lends to your failure, not to your success. There is no right way to exercise, and there are tons of gurus out there who promote different plans, you can find a method that works for you.

"I don't have time," is a complete lie. Time is created for things that are important, essential, and non-negotiable. When you began this journey, I'm pretty sure you told someone pre-op that you were "dedicated" to this journey.

Exercise is part of that.

Exercise is NON-NEGOTIABLE regardless of where you are. Here are some ways you can get exercise in, no matter what excuse you may have. I say this because there are chair exercises that you can find on YouTube if you're confined to your bed or chair.

You can move, and there are personal trainers online who design exercise programs just for you. Take to YouTube and type in "chair exercises," or "exercises for extreme obesity." I promise you that no matter where you are, there is a place for you to start.

If you are able, set yourself up to do three 10-minute walks per day, do one in the morning, one at lunch, and one in the evening. Whether you can get it in all at once, or whether you need to break it up for time reasons, this is a great way to start out and increase the time or intensity as you go.

When I started my workout routine, I literally walked around my house with my Fitbit on to track my time and my steps. Everyone will have different goals; however, the personal trainer at my surgeon's office recommended I get up to 10,000 steps a day by the time I had surgery.

You may want to ask your surgeon when you are ready for exercise. Each doctor will give specific medical advice, depending on the medical situation of the patient.

For individuals who are bedridden or in a wheelchair, you'll have a different set of recommendations or requirements. For individuals who are mobile, check and see how frequently your surgeon/physician wants you to get up and move around right after surgery.

Three months after surgery, my surgeon, and personal trainer recommended that I begin weight training. If you don't have a gym membership, try some YouTube videos and resistance bands.

Also, for individuals who may have trouble with knees, hips, or are wheelchair-bound, I recommend the chair workouts on YouTube. Anyone can get a good workout, no matter what!

Plan to get in at least three strength training workouts and three cardio workouts per week. Break it up in your day, and start small if you cannot do 30 minutes all at once, or if you don't have the time as noted above. Currently, I am training for 60–75 minutes at a time and work out 5–6 days per week. Many WLS patients can do this once they build up to it. Go at your own pace and add it as part of your day.

When you start small and increase the time by 5 minutes per day each week, you'll see what a difference it makes to your stamina, your mood, and to your endurance. Use an exercise tracker or fitness log to help you track your progress and your feelings. When you start to see how exercise impacts your mood positively, you'll be happy you started. Exercise will be a welcome habit of your new routine.

This is also an opportunity to take a "no excuses" approach to exercise. Whether you feel like it or not, you've got to move to be successful long term.

Take the First Step by Ripping off the Band-Aid …

Just do it, don't think about it!

"The future depends on what we do in the present." – Mahatma Gandhi

Stopping the "Do It Tomorrow" Attitude

Dealing with procrastination is a real issue.

Many of the WLS patients I've worked with talk about exercise as part of their desires and then don't follow through. They plan to act, they talk about wanting to act, and then, they don't act. They struggle with excuses and focus on a lack of time instead of creating time. This is purely a mindset issue because, at any point in time, you can decide to do something differently.

You may say, "No, really, I don't have time."

The thing is, we are all given the same amount of time in a day. We all have 24 hours, and what you do with it is up to you. Therefore, when people say they don't have time, the truth is, exercise, or meal planning, or whatever the activity may be, is purely not a priority.

Being someone who has been on the other side of this and found myself full of excuses. I realized, that when I made excuses at the time I made them, I sincerely felt that I did not have the time. I was not making it up.

Looking back, I recognize, had the task been important enough to me, I could've found a way to make it happen. That's the biggest difference between achievers and non-achievers, it's whether they want to find a way to make it happen, or whether they succumb to their HABIT of making excuses.

Notice here that I said the HABIT of excuses. Excuses are not always conscious decisions.

They are habits.

"When you do what you've always done, you'll get what you've always gotten." – Tony Robbins

This is an opportunity to dive deep into why you're making the excuse, so that you can overcome it and move past it.

Today is the day you make things happen, not tomorrow.

So often I'll hear people say, "I'll do it tomorrow," or "I'll begin tomorrow."

Tomorrow has its own actions. Today is the day that you create your tomorrow. Today is the day that you plant the seeds to reap the rewards.

If you do not act today, you will be in the same exact boat tomorrow. Therefore, today is the most important day that you have, because tomorrow will likely be the same until you do something today.

This may be a complex notion; however, when it was shared years ago with me by a meditation instructor, it hit me. I would put off things because of the uncomfortable feeling, surrounding doing them at the moment. I quickly realized that inaction produced more inaction, and action produces more action … which produces results.

If you want results, start taking action, for action begins with you. This may sound silly, but no one can walk two miles for you. Only you can do that. This is your journey, your goal, your life.

If you want to reap the harvest of tomorrow, seeing yourself thinner in the mirror, start acting today so you can produce those results tomorrow. Your actions happen today so you CAN reap those rewards in the future. Another way to say this is that you would not expect your employer to pay you today for work you'll do two weeks from now. It just doesn't work that way, so why would exercise or any other example?

Emotional Struggle with "Not Doing Things"
Procrastination and Fear of Success / Fear of Failure

I hear people share that they don't know why they "CANNOT" get themselves to do things.

Quite often I'll hear, "What's wrong with me? Why can't I just do it?"

Most often, the reason you are not acting has to do with a subconscious fear. It could be your fear of failure, fear of success, fear of "not good enough," or any other fear that once you act on it, you'll feel as though you are moving outside your comfort zone. This becomes very uncomfortable.

This is where the self-saboteur comes in. While there is a very big part of you that wants to change, there is another part of you that is very comfortable staying the same, and that part of you is likely fear-based.

Will people like me if I change?

What if people are jealous of me?

What if people think I'm hot shit when I get thin?

What if I become thinner than my sister and that might upset my family system?

What if I like myself as a thin person?

I may have to step up to the plate and people will have higher expectations of me.

What if people have higher expectations of me? What if I let them down?

What if I let myself down?

The thoughts are rampant. The fear of failure is ever present.

The fear of success is equally present because what if you can't live up to what you see for yourself?

This is all subconscious emotional gunk. Some theorists refer to this being "ego" as well. The ego keeps you safe by helping you stick within your comfort zone because when you expand outside your comfort zone, it's a place of unknowns.

Therefore, your ego does its best to mitigate disaster by giving you tons of reasons why you don't want to do something. This way you'll stay safe and warm inside your space of comfort. You and I both know that this type of comfort zone is not healthy, and when you grow beyond the egoic fears, you can transform your mind, your body, and your life.

Stop acting on autopilot, it's time for you to get back in control of your life.

You'll hear me talking a lot about autopilot behaviors. Most people live on autopilot because it's comfortable. It's a habit. It's what you've always done. It's what you've always known.

That doesn't make it good for you. Just because someone smokes for 20 years without cause, doesn't make it healthy. This is the same thing with eating behaviors and not exercising. Autopilot behaviors are subconscious habitual behaviors that are ingrained in your brain and in your behaviors.

When you start acting consciously, it may be uncomfortable at first because everything you are doing is different. However, just as if you were to learn to write with your non-dominant hand, at first it would be awkward and uncomfortable, but the more you did it, the easier it would get.

Your brain is built of neuropathways that are like highways. When you brush your teeth, this behavior started when you were a child. So, it's been ingrained in your brain to brush your teeth daily, a certain way, at a certain time. Likely when you wake up or go to bed, your rituals for morning or evening are on autopilot.

You probably don't even have to think about it because when you wake up, you walk to the bathroom and begin your morning routine. Your routine is already programmed in your brain as a habit and the neuropathways are programmed.

When you reject the old patterns of autopilot, you are transforming your mindset because you're altering your brain's program and reprogramming your subconscious mind. Likewise, you're building new neuropathways within your brain that support the new positive behaviors that you want to create in your life.

As you do this frequently, day in and day out, you'll create new habits over time that will help you live a successful and healthy life following weight loss surgery. Then this becomes the new pathways that you want your brain to take, causing a ripple effect of new positive behaviors.

Getting yourself to just do it

Getting started is one of the biggest issues my clients have trouble with because of the pattern of procrastination and then there is fear. The truth is once you get started, it's easy to gain momentum. But first, you must BEGIN.

The process of getting started does not have to be that difficult. The key to getting started is to stop thinking about getting started and to avoid overanalyzing the situation or the plan. Just do it.

Remember that old Nike commercial? "Just Do It" was the slogan. This is similar. The more you think about something, the more time your brain must find reasons and excuses for you NOT to do it. So instead of thinking about it, just act and get moving.

Taking a stand for your plan

I can't tell you how often I've worked with individuals who have given me excuses for why they haven't taken action. The truth is, if we want something bad enough, we create the time for it. How many times would the former you have gone through a drive-through and sat there for 10 plus minutes waiting for your order?

We will spend the time on something that is valuable to us. Likewise, if you want to go for a walk, you'll find the time or carve out time in your day to make it happen.

It begins with small steps. This is where you take a stand for yourself and recognize that inaction is the same as falling victim to your excuses. We are the creators of our excuses and likewise, we can be the banisher of them as well.

You got surgery for a reason. You made the decision to change your life. This is a decision that you make not ONCE, but every single day with the actions you take. So, take a stand for yourself, for your life, and recognize that it's not the one BIG decision to have surgery that changes your life, but the smaller decisions you make every day that really make an impact over time.

As I write this, I think back to writing another portion of this book where I discuss Darren Hardy's book *The Compound Effect*. This book helped me see that what we do over time compounds and creates our outcome. As we are creatures of habit, we tend to do things over and over and over. Consequently, I focus so heavily on sharing mindset shifts that help you to create habit shifts long term.

When you do something just once, it can help you to do it over, and over, and over again. Likewise, if you only do something once, it won't give you as big of an impact. If you were to go through the drive-through and order a burger once, there will not be much of an impact on your overall life or health.

However, if you start to go daily, or a few times a week, creating a habit of going through the drive-through and ordering burgers, you'll begin to see a shift in your habits, your waistline, your weight, and in how you feel because this has created a bigger impact on your life.

If you were to walk only once, you may not see a big impact. BUT, if you began walking 15 minutes per day, every day, or several times per week, you'll start to see a difference in how you feel, you may see that your muscles are getting toned, that you have more stamina, your mood is elevated, and that you feel healthier overall.

When you take a stand for yourself, it starts with that initial step and requires you to reignite the fire within you again, and again, and again so that you can build the habits and see the long-term results.

Dear Motivation, where oh where are you?

Motivation is not something to be found. It's something that you develop within. I've shared articles on this topic and take a stand that motivation is not something that you sit around or wait for, it's something that you get up and get.

Wait, wait, wait … WHAT!?!?

Most people believe that motivation is something that you wait on, like inspiration. Motivation is not a bus, it's not coming around if you sit on a bench outside your house. Motivation comes from within, and it's like a fire that you light within yourself. It's something that is built one step at a time, over time. Are you ready to get motivated??

Chapter Journaling Prompts

What will it take for me to create a plan?

What are the fears that pop up for me?

What are the most important steps for me to focus on?

What are my weight loss / physical goals?

What have I noticed in my mindset that I recognize needs shifting?

What steps can I take today to move toward my goals?

Chapter 4

Following the Plan – Decision, Commitment & Consistency

"When you only do what is easy, life will be hard. When you do what is hard, life will be easy." – T. Harv Eker

The Practical Parts of the Plan – Planning ahead as discussed in chapter 3 and now implementing the plan.

"Will it be easy? Nope. Will it be worth it? Absolutely!" – Author unknown

Staying the course will help you to be consistent over the long term. If you know what you'll be eating, it will help you shave time off the process. You'll shop faster, you'll cook easier, and it will work like a well-oiled machine.

Of course, there will be days and times when your schedule gets messed up and things get off track. That is just life. However, you've got to plan for that too!

What? Plan for that? How?

I know ... I know, it sounds crazy.

I've had people say that to me before. How can I plan for the unexpected?

On any given week, things are going to get moved around. Expect that and plan around it. Planning is about planning for what you expect, and what you don't expect.

Your plan is your greatest asset because it puts you in control of your greatest weapon for success and at the same time your greatest saboteur: yourself.

Jennifer is a 42-year-old mother of two. She has struggled with her weight most of her life, going up and down on the scale like a yo-yo, in her words. She struggled with losing weight, sharing that nothing worked for her.

In my clinical assessment of her, I asked her what she had tried to lose weight. Like me, she had tried everything; however, when she shared what she tried and when she tried it, her timeline was a bit different. See, Jennifer would not stay on a plan very long. In fact, she shared that she had trouble staying on any specific plan longer than 3–4 weeks.

Clearly, this was a big red flag, because she wasn't committed to any of the plans she tried. So how was she planning to commit to lifestyle change following bariatric surgery?

This is where we dug deeper into her story. Jennifer really wanted more choices and got bored with eating and didn't want to be tied down to a single plan because she said she felt controlled. When we included more variety into her meals, she felt more in control and comfortable with the choices available to her. The thing is, Jennifer decided to commit to a plan and then became frustrated with it.

People change their minds every day. This is not the issue. However, many people have trouble committing to things when things get tough. With Jennifer, we could unravel her emotional ties to food and help her get back on track quickly.

For others, it's not so simple. Commitment to a plan can be severely uncomfortable for people, because the plan can get boring, and food may be a source of excitement for them, especially when many options are available. This is where commitment can become a sticky issue.

Following your plan after lifestyle surgery is what will help you to stay successful in the long run, yet life is full of twists and turns. You'll have days where meetings go long, and evenings where the kids have track practice, ballet, or you have a late PTA meeting. There will be days and nights where cooking seems impossible and picking up food on the way home seems so much easier. I get it, and I'm living it with you.

Having a plan does not mean never picking up food that is quick, it means not picking up fast food, which is totally different. You can find, pick up, and/or make healthy options that are quick if you know what they are. Additionally, anticipating the hectic craziness that is life in advance will help you stay on track even more.

My client Melanie shared that life is always throwing her curveballs, and it's hard for her to cook. She travels for work, is a full-time mom of two, and is struggling to manage her household, and life in general, all while trying to stay "on plan" after bariatric surgery. So instead of having a static plan for Melanie, we created a fluid plan that worked with her schedule, her family, her type of meals (bari-friendly), and for her lifestyle.

Just because you've had bariatric surgery does not mean life stops. You will still be busy. You will still experience crazy days. The difference is planning for and anticipating how well you can stay on track during these times instead of returning to excuses about how it's so hard.

Eating on a plan helps you to lose the weight, feel better, and with that, there is a greater sense of accomplishment. When you return to old habits and use lifestyle as an excuse, you are living in the OLD VERSION of you, not the new upgraded version of yourself.

This is where your commitment comes in. This is developed through your mindset.

"Stay committed to your decisions, but stay flexible in your approach." – Tony Robbins

For some individuals losing weight will be easy because they will stick to the plan. For others, they will have to work at it despite having bariatric surgery. This is where the mindset piece comes in.

As you commit to the process, you begin to build a new mindset dedicated and focused on the new habits. However, if you slide back into old habits, you'll likely end up in regain. Hence, the mindset piece is essential, because awareness is the mother of change.

When you begin to see that you are sliding backward, you can catch yourself. However, if you have no awareness into your behaviors, then you'll likely fall back without awareness and wonder how you got there to begin with. This is why we are here, to help you become aware, stay aware, and be the pilot of your life.

You've been on autopilot too long, and it's time for you to take back control and live consciously. Who is really driving the bus of your life? Most likely, your subconscious mind.

When you put your conscious mind in control, and you take conscious actions and build new habits over time, you then reprogram your mind all while taking back control indefinitely.

Prior to surgery, I experienced struggle after struggle. If my entire life was not revolved around focusing on making weight loss happen, it wasn't happening. Furthermore, even when the weight loss behaviors had become the central focus of my life, I still wasn't losing much weight. This left me frustrated and disillusioned with the entire process.

Having bariatric surgery changed my life because it made massive weight loss possible for me. At first, the weight loss was easy, and this felt so good. I know this is true for many of my clients and other bariatric surgery patients everywhere.

I also know that having bariatric surgery is not a "one and done" action. After surgery, there is a mandatory lifestyle change that must occur for people to get to their goal weight and to sustain the long-term weight loss. When people return to old habits and make poor choices, they are bound for regain over time. The research suggests that individuals who are better at self-monitoring such as weighing themselves regularly and keeping records (food journals, and meal plans for example), are much more likely to maintain their weight (Odom, 2016).

Additionally, it is also predicted that those are most likely to gain weight after bariatric surgery are those who have a lack of control when it comes to food urges and those who have issues with alcohol or drugs (Odom, 2016).

Therefore, making a commitment to yourself and this new bariatric lifestyle is CRITICAL.

Why would you go and get a $20,000+ surgery to change your life, and then not follow the recommended plan afterward?

I believe this behavior is because of three main things: a lack of commitment, a lack of consistency, and the emotional underbelly that many avoid because it's uncomfortable. Within this chapter, we'll cover commitment and consistency, and in subsequent chapters, I'll go over the emotional components of weight loss surgery patients, and how to deal with the emotional piece.

This may not come up for you right away, and instead, it comes up after your six-month- or one-year mark. This is because most people get started like a racehorse right out of the gate, going strong. Then, they reach what I call "the messy middle."

You get into the weeds, into the thick of it. You get tempted around foods. You may return to old behaviors, or one step at a time, start with a chip here, or an afternoon non-plan approved snack there, or you have a roll before dinner just because they brought them to the table ... and then ... BOOM! Before you know it, you'll be asking yourself how you ended up with 45 lb. of regain.

I'm sharing this because I've seen it happen, and I'm writing this book, so you can be fully aware and awake to how it happens. It does not happen overnight. It happens gradually.

It's time for you to stay on track by staying committed to the intentions and plans you set for yourself each and every week. When you are committed week after week, month after month, even when the WLS honeymoon is over, then you'll see the long-term success.

This is where flexibility comes in. Everyone has a honeymoon period and for just about everyone, the honeymoon ends. Creating flexibility within your plans allows for greater awareness and greater control over your life and choices.

Most recently my client Wendy, a nurse, told me that she struggled with eating hospital cafeteria food when she was famished and had forgotten to plan. She would go for the chicken fingers, avoiding the fries, but still felt horrible that she resorted to fried foods.

We discussed her non-negotiables for eating in the cafeteria and came up with four solid choices that she could choose from when this was her last resort. Having her list in hand the next three times she had to eat in the cafeteria helped her to feel more in control because she didn't allow the other options to even enter her mind.

She had created flexibility in her plan and was clear on her non-negotiables. Fried chicken, grilled cheese, and fries were among her non-negotiables and on her not-eating list, while grilled chicken, high protein yogurt, a turkey burger patty (no bun), and hard-boiled eggs on a mini salad were among her top bariatric-approved food choices for cafeteria dining.

She planned even when she forgot to plan and created flexibility within her unplanned plan for maximum effectiveness.

Building Consistency = Creating New Behaviors & Habits

"We are what we repeatedly do; success is not an action but a habit." – Aristotle

"So, how do I build consistency?"

For many of us in this "instant gratification" society, we get bored with plans, doing the same thing over and over, and repeating events. Yet, that's what consistency is.

Consistency literally means "conformity in the application of something." Therefore, when you are committed to your plan, you are doing it over and over and over. You are meal planning weekly, you are sticking to your exercise schedule, you are checking off your water intake, you are taking your supplements daily, and so on.

This means you are creating new behaviors, which become your new habits over time. However, it does not have to be rote or boring. You can make your plan exciting to keep things interesting.

The "messy middle" is where things get tough. It is usually the same place where "all hell breaks loose." You cannot give up at this point even if you feel like you want to or need to. What you do need is to reassess what's working for you and what's not.

This also goes back to being flexible.

No one starts off their plan and says, "You know what? I'm going to start off great, hit a wall, get bored, get tied up with work, forget to do my meal plan, feel like a failure, throw my hands up in the air and then get so frustrated with myself that my behavior will fizzle out."

No one plans for that.

That's no one's intentions, yet that's exactly what happens most of the time. Life happens.

Frustration. Anxiety. Bosses. Stress. Jobs. Kids. Spouses. Family. School. Money. Parents. Life.

You can make an interpretation however you wish, looking at these words as they pertain to the specifics in your life, and although I may not know you personally, I know you.

I know where you get stuck because we all get stuck in the same places.

My client Leslie started off after surgery fantastic. She lost 72 lb. in 6 months and was on fire with her progress. She continued to do great through her 9th month when she switched job's and her whole schedule changed.

She was a nurse used to working day shift and moved to an afternoon/evening shift where she didn't return home until after 1 AM. She got up later, ate later, and as a result, started eating later in general.

This would not have been an issue, but she started eating a snack right after she got home. The snack then turned into a meal, and then she ended up gaining back 13 lb. within a two-month period, not understanding what happened.

When we started working together, we unraveled her eating history and recognized that she had done two things beyond changing her work schedule. First, she stopped meal planning because she wasn't at home in the evenings to cook for her family, and did not see the point. Secondly, she started grazing instead of eating her three solid meals as a post-WLS patient.

When we went over her plan, we adjusted the meal plan for her family, so she could eat the same foods they ate. We also created more flexibility in her plan so that if her shift changed, she would be able to eat early enough that it did not affect her sleep schedule, and so she would not get super hungry and graze.

The focus of our plan was on flexibility and changing things up as her schedule change.

Rigidity and a one-size-fits-all approach doesn't work when life is ever changing. Revaluate your plan frequently so you can adjust as needed. This is a very necessary component of staying on track and when building consistency with your meal plans, eating plans, and for achieving your goals.

Creating Motivation

"Don't watch the clock; do what it does. Keep going." – Sam Levenson

Motivation is a very important part of following your plan.

People often ask me where they get their motivation from, as if motivation is a magic pill, potion, or answer. There is no magic answer regarding motivation. The truth is, we create our own motivation out of what we desire.

Your level of commitment is equal to what you determine to be a non-negotiable in your life. Your level of commitment to something determines your motivation.

However, the barrier to your motivation is the present moment.

When you see something that you crave in the present, you may forget the future picture of yourself that you have longed to see, because the pull toward the food is much more exciting than something that may or may not happen within the next 6–12 months.

When there is uncertainty of whether something will happen, your brain seeks certainty. So, therefore, you may reach out for the food because that is right in front of you, and it is more certain that what may or may not happen six months from now.

However, what you do today impacts your tomorrow, and your tomorrow's tomorrow. So that one piece of chocolate today may not make an impact, but the chocolate you ate yesterday, the piece you eat today, tomorrow, and the next day and the day after that will have a greater impact over time.

This is how your brain works prior to surgery, you look for the most certain thing right now: the food. However, after surgery, your stomach is smaller, and while some people have more self-control per meal, the grazing behaviors get out of control.

Even now, close your eyes and take a mental picture yourself after losing all the weight.

How do you feel emotionally?

How do you feel physically in your body?

Are you more flexible?

Do you have more stamina or endurance?

What can you do now with this new body that you could not do before?

What do you want to do now that you haven't been able to do before?

Doesn't this excite you and exhilarate you?

Most people are excited about STARTING a plan and seeing their RESULTS. However, the middle is typically more difficult and often referred to as being like "moving through sludge." You get bored, you wonder if you'll ever hit your goals.

Success depends on you moving through the sludge, on a step-by-step basis even when it feels hard, impossible, the desire isn't there. Your action means everything.

There are days you won't "feel" like it. I get it.

Even when you feel like you are moving backward, it's better than not moving at all. Also, you've got to get moving and act on your plan instead of staying stagnant.

Start moving forward by recommitting yourself to your plan. Then add some strategy. What gets you going? What do you get excited about?

"People often say that motivation doesn't last. Well, neither does bathing – that's why we recommend it daily." – Zig Ziglar

Creating motivation within yourself and for yourself is the core of mindset work.

Each morning when I wake up, I grab my journal and I write down 5 things I'm grateful for. Then I write things that I'd like to see happen in my life. Then I sent intentions for the day, such as a mini to-do list.

Then I focus on how I will feel once I reach my goals (thinking big picture).

Then I focus on how I will feel once I reach complete my daily intention list (smaller picture / smaller accomplishments).

Then I focus on how my short-term daily list helps me get closer to my bigger picture goals.

Then I pull it all together.

I also use visualizations, EFT, and other exercises that I share in chapter 6 as part of my mindset work.

Using these tools will help you to stay motivated because you are creating more certainty by taking consistent action.

Just like Olympic athletes prepare for a game, a race, or a championship, through doing mindset work, you are preparing your own mind for success.

You may not have done mindset work in the past; however, mindset work is the key to getting motivated and staying motivated. Just like Zig Ziglar says, we bath daily. Why would we expect motivation to last any longer than a day? It doesn't. Therefore, by cultivating a daily practice, you can ensure you harness the power of motivation to your benefit to keep you going, even when life takes you off course.

Focus on your mindset, take consistent action, persevere and the results will follow.

Here are some additional exercises for accessing the motivation within.

~ Strategy 1: Challenge yourself

Are you someone who likes to win? If yes, create a game where you challenge yourself to get 4 out of 6 days of exercise in. Or challenge yourself to plan and stick to it.

Then keep score of how often you completed the activities you said you would do and then check your progress.

This is an exciting way to see your progress and also notice all the things you're doing toward your goals.

~ Strategy 2: Keep a success journal of your accomplishments

Maybe you've gone from lifting 20 lb. to 30 lb. at the gym.

Maybe you can run 25 miles without stopping.

Maybe you decided to apply for a new job.

Maybe you turned down doughnuts at the company meeting last week.

Maybe you stood up for yourself in a heated situation.

Whatever they may be, you've got to track them to remember that they happened.

These are amazing accomplishments that show your progress, which are not about weight at all.

The reason for this is that at your LOWEST emotional point, you won't remember your successes, and instead your mind will align with all the crappy stuff that has happened, is happening, or that you are projecting to happen. This is because your mind is programmed around fear and fear-based thinking.

When you are having a rough day, feel bloated, or get on the scale and you may have gained a pound, your brain will go find all the ways you are a failure instead of reminding you of all the ways you are awesome.

When you go into full freak-out negative self-talk mode feeling that you have gone south, having a success journal that you can reflect on will help you gain perspective and shift you back to the appropriate course.

This will help you reignite your motivation and refocus your attention on what you want most, to continue your path of weight loss and keep it off for good.

~ Strategy 3: Remember WHY you started

Reflect on how you got here. You may not know "how" you got as big as you did, but when you remember what you want, this will help you shift gears.

This is not a strategy that can be rushed. Take your time and reflect on your biggest desires. Go beyond the weight and look at the significance that the long-term weight loss will bring you.

What are your reasons for "WHY" you began this journey?

Cultivating Success through Perseverance

"You just can't beat the person who never gives up." – Babe Ruth

The old you may have given up; however, the new you is a fighter.

The new you is ready to take on the world.

So why would you ever give up?

MINDSET!

Again, the middle is super messy.

Perseverance is key. This requires a keen shift in mindset, so you can and will stay on course.

Jim is 55 and had 178 lb. to lose. He had lost about 127 lb., and he hit a stall. He knew stalls were bound to happen, so it was expected. However, when he ended up in a stall for nearly 4 months, he began to panic. He wondered what "more" he could do to get back on the "losing train" and his mindset was at a point where he felt he was failing.

The truth was, Jim wasn't failing, and in fact, he was right on track. He went over his meal plan with his dietitian, we discussed his emotions, and he had his labs checked by his doctor. He was right on point. However, his panic was created by his inner fear that he could not move past his stall.

We discussed his fears and all the emotions that came up as well as using many of the tools suggested in chapter 6, to help him move through the stall. However, in addition to the tools and techniques, Jim was sure that he would continue to his goal. His perseverance was key. He continued to eat on-plan, got enough sleep, and exercised regularly. After a period of another two months, Jim started losing again, this time having a 5-lb. drop when he checked the scale.

The point here is not to get obsessive, or overly focused on the stalls, but to reflect regularly on your plan of action, as well as your follow-through, but continuing to persevere no matter what.

Perseverance also is important when life takes a left turn. We are all human and no one is immune to "life happens." However, it's never about what happens in life, and typically all in how we respond to it, which is all about the mindset.

Therefore, cultivating a mindset of perseverance and having non-negotiables are essential for the long-term success of a WLS patient.

Chapter 5

Building Your Support System

Everyone needs support after bariatric surgery. You're not alone, even when you may feel like it. There are so many emotional and physical changes after WLS, there are days you will need more support than others. It's about knowing who you can count on, and who you will surround yourself with.

We'll dig deeper into relationship issues in chapter 8, but for now, let's focus on where you can get support, and the importance of getting the help you need following surgery.

Knowing who, what, and when to ask for help is essential in being successful on your journey. This chapter will cover the various places/people you can reach out to for added support. It can come in the form of another person, self-guided support, or even professional support.

Never be afraid to ask for help. It could be the difference in your success or failure.

Your Support System and Asking for Help

You might be too shy to ask for help. You might feel like a burden if you are asking for help. Or you might believe that others are too busy for you.

If you were like me, with relatives that were the food police, you are REALLY unlikely to ask for help, especially if you feel they are watching your every move. I've had clients that shared with me that their family has made comments like "Are you allowed to eat that?" or "What would your doctor say if he saw you eating that?"

Also, it could be likely that you may have people in your life who believe you've taken the "easy" way out. Please note that bariatric surgery is NOT the easy way out. As we've gotten deeper into this, I hope you see that this is a lifestyle change and requires your commitment to the plan and staying on track through consistency for you to achieve the long-term results.

Don't let those comments hurt or offend you. Those comments come from a place of ignorance, and although it seems like they may be said out of a place of malice, they are most often not.

However, this time it is different. Yet, you also need to understand that just because they cut your stomach, don't think your head, emotions, or mindset will change because honestly, they don't. At least, not until you start working on those components, which is why you are here reading this book.

You and I both know that you definitely want change inside and out. You don't want to stay the same old person and you want to know how to ask for help and guidance so that you don't end up harboring the food police again.

You want genuine support that will guide you toward success, not toward shame, blame, and guilt. Am I right?

When you hear those comments, take a deep breath in, and forgive the person spouting them (if you can!). You know in your heart of hearts that you had this surgery to save your life, and you are reading this book to get a handle on the post-surgical behavioral changes.

You are here for a reason and you don't need additional negativity. You need support, love, and people who will help to lift you up, so you can stay on track, not those who tear you down.

With that said, there will be those people. It's up to you if you decide to cut them loose from your life. You might even have a friend, spouse, or another person in your life who is jealous of your weight loss, or is a serial enabler.

You know this type, the person who makes brownies the second you told them you were on a diet. You know who I'm talking about. Then they act innocently, and then behind your back, they are plotting. If you've had an honest conversation with them with open communication and this has not helped, you might want to look at releasing them from your life.

It's a difficult decision to make; however, as you've begun this journey for yourself, there will be people who are not ready to be on that journey with you, and that's OK.

You also want to begin living your life, having fun, and doing things that make you happy. There will be some people who you really need support from, and then there are other outlets you need purely for the social benefit.

Here are six different ways to gain support after WLS/bariatric surgery:

❖ Get a Journal – You are your own buddy

Writing is not for everyone and some people may find it difficult to be their own support system. I get it. Journaling is not for everyone. I've had some clients who absolutely detest journaling and that is OK. Others find it very enjoyable and insightful.

Many of my very successful clients keep a daily journal where they write down their emotions while keeping a food diary. This is great because they are tracking both their food intake and their emotional status. Sometimes overeating or grazing occurs due to emotional issues, so when you pair them together, it can be a huge awareness that helps you grow.

Writing is also a great way to get out of your head. Many of my clients and other WLS patients I've talked to discuss how journaling has helped them stay on track in the long run because when they hit an emotional upset, they go to the journal to write it out.

This will help you get it out of your head and onto the paper. It's a great way to get in touch with your emotions and process your emotions. Even when you are not sure what they might be, the journaling process can help you identify feelings you did not know you had, and find the feelings that you may be avoiding, all through getting clear with yourself by putting pen to paper.

❖ Phone a Friend or Family Member

Having someone you can call is always a great plan. No person is an island and we all need social support. Calling a dear friend can help you get out of a funk and remind you of what you are working toward. Whenever there may be a struggle in any area of your life, your friends are there to go to bat for you.

Whether you call a dear friend or family member, having someone in your corner is the goal. Confiding in someone you can trust helps you to release the emotions you may have pent up inside. Talking it out is always helpful because friends are great at support and help us see things from another perspective.

Call the friends or family members who you know will be most supportive and offer the soundest advice. Try to stay away from the negative family members who want to tout "I told you so" nonsense, or want to lecture you about your new lifestyle. Also, be patient with those who don't understand, and refocus your attention back on your own needs when you need support.

Reach out to those who are supportive and allow your support system to help you when you need it. In other words, allow yourself to be helped. Sometimes bariatric patients feel "guilty" for asking family and friends for help. This is a great opportunity to further build your relationships, so allow them to help and please, please, please, do not feel bad about it.

❖ Attend a Support Group Meeting or Join an Online Support Group

Support groups are great because they are typically filled with people just like you, going through similar circumstances. Support groups offer a lot of value because you can share things that the group can relate to and you feel that you are part of something bigger.

Look for support groups in your area, and they are typically offered at WLS surgical centers and hospitals. You can also create your own support group if you know enough people struggling with similar issues.

You can also attend our FREE online private support group on Facebook: **Bariatric Mindset Mavens**

❖ Get NEW Bariatric Friends

Surround yourself with people who are on a similar path. This is like the suggestion above; however, when you can talk to and hang out with people who are on a similar journey, then you can support each other through the process.

You may even find people at your support group or through online means. There are many online forums and support groups that allow people to speak freely about their journey, and is a good place to ask questions, get answers, and talk to other people who are experiencing similar things.

Also, having people who are like-minded will help you expand your mindset after WLS because they will likely have similar wins and struggles. This way you can help each other grow.

❖ Learn Something New / Expand Your Social Circle

Taking a class or course is a great way to expand your social circle and your knowledge base. This is also a great way to meet new friends and get yourself out there. If you are someone who may have been housebound or not as active in the past, getting out is a good way to get yourself moving and engaging with others.

This is also a great way to cook healthier food and take a cooking class that may help you excel on your bariatric journey. You can take a spin class at the local gym, or learn scrapbooking.

Search online in your local area to see if there are meetups that may be of interest to you, or check out your local community colleges or university for "community" classes that are open to all individuals in the community.

Recently, one of my clients took a painting class and met three new friends. Another client of mine decided to take pottery and photography classes. These are just examples of activities to get involved in and meet new people.

The individuals you meet will not be your initial support system; however, when your mind is busy and your body is active, you're transforming into the new you: the person who lives his/her life actively, not passively.

❖ Find a Therapist/Counselor/Coach

You don't need to have mental health issues or feel that you are "severe" to see a therapist or counselor. Anyone can see a therapist or counselor to help them move forward in their lives.

A coach is a good option with regard to accountability. One caveat is that not all coaches are certified, and the coaching field is largely unregulated. Therefore, I use extreme caution in recommending you seek out a coach because, by and large, many coaches are not qualified to deal with bariatric/WLS issues.

Many so-called health coaches don't have the psychological background knowledge that counselors/therapists do, and if they are not certified, please be careful.

Make sure that whoever you choose – therapist, counselor, or coach – that you have thoroughly vetted them to see if they are qualified to work with you and your situation.

In my experience, personality and connection matters. Most people select a therapist/counselor through insurance; however, you'll see your therapist or counselor more frequently than you'll see your doctor. You'll be sharing more intimate details than you'd share with your doctor, so find someone who you resonate with, and can help you grow.

When I saw the eating disorders specialist, I only chose her based on her clinical qualifications. She was not an insurance provider either, and so I remember thinking that this was an investment in myself. However, my big mistake was that I only focused on her credentials, not our connection.

Not too long into the process, I realized that I really needed a professional who understood my goals, my issues, what I wanted to accomplish, and someone who was both qualified and a good personality fit with me to help me get to where I needed to go.

Sitting on the other side of the couch, as I am a therapist/counselor, and coach, not everyone jives with me, and that's OK. Not everyone will, and I don't carry the expectation that everyone will like my treatment style.

In fact, I prefer only to work with people who want to work with me and who are excited to work with me, and usually, those same people are the ones that I'm excited to work with as well. This is how the therapeutic relationship is built. There are people you will build a connection with, and others that you will not. This is life.

That's why there are a million counselors/therapists, psychologists, and coaches out there. As bariatric patients, we want to work with someone who speaks to us, who will understand us, and who will push us outside of our little comfort zone box to help us grow.

Don't be fooled to think that just because someone is on your insurance panel that they will have what it takes to serve you, meet your needs, and help you grow. They may be fully qualified, have all the correct letters behind their name, be on your insurance panel, be a great person, and still, they might not be a good fit for you; and that is OK too.

However, if you are choosing a therapist/counselor solely because of your insurance, and IF they are not a good fit, you may be in therapy longer because when it's not a good fit, it's just not a good fit. Therefore, the therapeutic relationship or coaching relationship, whatever you choose, should be paramount in your decision-making process.

Finding someone right for you is important. This is deep work, and you'll want someone to guide you on this journey who is there to support you, guide you, challenge the negative internal beliefs, and to help you see things that you don't see yourself. This person is there to help you unpack your baggage and get rid of it.

Would you want someone to help you that you just are "meh" about seeing on a weekly or biweekly basis? This is YOUR LIFE! This is your JOURNEY! Find someone awesome and begin.

Additionally, about insurance. I know for many people insurance is the way to go because of financial concerns. There are many qualified out-of-network counselors/therapists who have sliding fee scales, who will create super-bills, so you can submit to try to get reimbursed through your insurance. It's also important to note that coaches are not insurance providers and those fees come fully out of pocket.

The point is, whether you choose an insurance provider or not, focus on your connection and you can't go wrong. The most important thing in the process is your growth and helping you reach your goals.

Whatever your choice, be committed to it for the right reasons for you, take the steps needed, and you will see the growth.

Chapter 6

Using Tools to Help You Grow

Within my private practice, I use various tools to help my clients achieve long-term weight loss success. Some of them I've already included in this book in other chapters.

You'll see activities on building awareness, practical tools such as creating a meal plan or exercise plan, and in subsequent chapters I give examples of how to get clarity on what you really want.

In this chapter, we'll be focusing on mindset work to help you shift your belief systems using tools that get you to remove limiting beliefs and old negative thinking patterns using a variety of techniques. I'll also include mindful eating and releasing the limiting beliefs that may have kept you stuck in old patterns.

As discussed previously, each of us has a conscious mind and subconscious mind, which are programmed differently. What you are conscious of, you can shift and change quickly.

Our subconscious beliefs are not so easily changed. Therefore, self-sabotage can come up because how can you change something you are not aware of?

Eating Mindfully

Mindful eating is important because pre-surgery most people have reported having autopilot eating behaviors. Mindful eating is an essential element of weight loss success because it helps individuals slow down and focus on the process of eating. For a few minutes, you are doing nothing else but eating. Try one of these mindful eating techniques and see if it makes a difference.

Many of my clients who have struggled with mindful eating at first typically have shame around eating in general. So, slowing down the eating can become stressful for them. This exercise makes eating an enjoyable process where you can sit and enjoy your food by slowing down and tasting it.

One client of mine told me that he was so used to "inhaling" his food. And that sitting down, and slowing down, while eating was uncomfortable. I asked him to try it a few times and journal about his emotions. He felt the need to just "get the food down." His shame did not come out initially, and after examining his habits, it emerged.

Eating slowly became uncomfortable because he wasn't eating for his body, he was eating for his emotions, filling a void, and this kept him from truly experiencing and enjoying his food. The reason that slowing down and eating was uncomfortable was because he shared that enjoying the food made him feel guilty.

He had carried around so much shame about his weight that he told me he felt undeserving of eating, and that while he knew he had to eat, that if he ate fast, he could avoid feeling the shameful feelings that eating provided. This behavior was also followed by hours of avoiding eating, until he could eat alone, and then he would eat very quickly so no one would see him.

Another client, who had a similar behavior of inhaling food, shared that he had experienced a situation in childhood that if he didn't finish his food, it would be given to his siblings because there was not enough to go around.

Everyone's story about "why" they eat fast or why they struggle with slowing down will be different. Examine your story.

What comes up for you?

What resistance (if any) do you have to slowing down your eating process?

What urges do you feel when you are asked to put the fork down between bites?

What feelings come up when you are asked to chew your food more between bites?

List these answers out and reflect on them. This will provide insight into the deeper issues that may be continuing to come up for you in your eating routine and at meals.

Exercise 1: Mindful Eating

Sit down with your food and no other distractions (such as telephone, TV, or computer). Take a look at what is on your plate. Take a photo of it if you like. Then slowly and consciously take one bite at a time with time to put your fork down.

This process is about enjoying the food in front of you and tasting the different flavors that you are experiencing. Take conscious bites and chew your food at least 10 times before swallowing.

What do you notice about the taste?

What do you notice about the texture?

What do you notice about your thoughts/feelings?

Take a moment to reflect on the flavors you can taste in each bite. Do you sense something bitter, or sweet, or is it too salty, or not salty enough?

What flavors do you prefer?

After you've eaten, write down your observations in your journal and date it with today's date. Try this once per day for a week and notice the changes if any over the course of a week.

Many of the individuals I've worked with have noticed that when they do this exercise, they initially feel resistance to slowing down to eat, or eating without distractions. However, by the end of the week, they report that they feel more satiated, more satisfied with their food, and don't feel any urge to graze or overeat.

Try this for a week and track your progress.

What have you noticed?

What patterns have emerged?

What emotions have emerged?

What changes in your eating behaviors have emerged?

Exercise 2: Conscious Eating

If you don't like it, don't eat it. This does not mean run out and order cheeseburgers, but what I am saying is don't sit there at the dinner table and eat food that is not both nourishing and satisfying. One of my clients shared that she would mindlessly eat rolls or tortilla chips at the dinner table, and "didn't even really like them, but they were there," so she ate them.

The bariatric patient cannot afford to eat filler foods anymore; however, the reaching out of one's hand for the filler foods is a habit. Many of the people who I speak with that go after filler foods are struggling more with FOMO – the fear of missing out.

FOMO is a mental and emotional habit, not a physical need for food. Therefore, this is all about head hunger, and it's your mental or emotional state that wants to be satisfied, not your body.

I had a client who ate food simply to fill the urge. One specific time she shared that her friend made a crustless quiche, and she was hungry, so she ate it, but really did not like it. When she returned home, she noticed that she was still hungry because she was so dissatisfied with the quiche that she felt she HAD to eat something else.

This is another example of, "If you don't like it, don't eat it," and make other plans instead!! You are not a garbage disposal. If you don't like something, love yourself, and your body enough to say, "No, thank you," and find something that is both equally satisfying and nourishing.

This suggested exercise is about consciously eating foods that you like that are also within your plan. It's not about never eating certain foods again, but about being conscious about what you are putting into your body. I have clients who focus on protein first, eat on-plan regularly and will occasionally, have a single piece of chocolate. This satisfies them, and they move on.

Please take note that I said occasionally, and the word occasionally means: "At infrequent or irregular intervals; now and then." This does not mean once a day, or even once a week.

Remember that your patterns and habits dictate your results. Having ONE single piece of chocolate now and again is not prohibited, but it's important to know on a very personal level if you can handle this or if you can't. Some people struggle with eating just ONE of anything, while others can allow themselves to have a single piece and experience satisfaction.

Furthermore, if you don't like kale, don't eat it. Instead eat other vegetables you do like. Likewise, don't eat french fries because they are present in front of you. Eating consciously means eating for both taste and nutritional content. Using these two together can help you stay on track because you are making a conscious decision about what you are putting into your body. This process also may help guide you down a path of changing your taste buds as well.

Again, this process is not about deprivation, it's about being very conscious of your choices, of your behaviors, and of your habits. Your future you will thank you for it.

Journaling Prompts:

What are you more conscious about after trying this process?

What insight have you gained into your eating behaviors?

EFT

(Emotional Freedom Techniques)

What is EFT tapping? I get asked this a lot by individuals who have never experienced it before.

EFT or emotional freedom techniques is also known as "tapping" or "EFT tapping". EFT is an energy psychology technique and universal healing tool aimed at reducing limiting beliefs and that can provide impressive results for physical, emotional, and performance issues by tapping on the acupressure energy points on the surface of the skin.

EFT tapping helps to shift subconscious beliefs by focusing the mind on specific psychological problems or goals, thereby releasing them through the tapping process. Through the EFT tapping process, the brain's neuropathways are accessed, and subconscious beliefs and processes can be shifted quickly to help the user to change unwanted habits or behaviors, or to shift emotional states such as anxiety, fear, guilt, shame, or anger.

It also helps people in reprogramming the subconscious mind with new empowering beliefs that help people enhance their ability to succeed in their endeavors and enjoy life.

According to the Association for Comprehensive Energy Psychology, EFT is sometimes called "acupressure for the emotions." EFT, or "tapping," is a highly focused energy psychology method that rapidly releases the emotional impact of stressful or traumatic life events from the body-mind system.

As clients bring their attention to distressing memories and symptoms, practitioners walk them through a process of voicing specific statements while tapping on a series of acupuncture meridian points. This activation appears to reduce levels of stress while stimulating the processing of previously stuck emotions and habit patterns (ACEP, 2017).

I believe in this practice so much, because I've cleared so much negative energy and negative belief statements from my own mind. A few years ago, when I started using this with my own clients, we began to see incredible results instantaneously.

All of my clients reported feeling a decrease in cravings, a change in their behavior, and when they tapped during a period of feeling emotional eating triggers, they felt more in control of themselves, and the mental/emotional need for food would be released as a result of the tapping.

Of course, they were very clear on what they were tapping through, so once these beliefs were identified, they knew when to tap, how to tap, and what beliefs they needed to tap on so they could release them and move forward.

What's the Process? How Do I Do It?

The process of EFT tapping starts by identifying limiting beliefs, so they can be "tapped out" of your subconscious mind.

The second phase is to "tap out" the negative or limiting beliefs, or troublesome emotional state through tapping through the points on one's body.

The third phase is to reframe the beliefs and to write down new empowering beliefs that we want to reprogram into the subconscious mind.

The way we do this is by tapping in a specific pattern through the tapping points. It's a good idea if you are alone when you do this because sometimes people may not understand what you are doing, and it can thoroughly distract your process.

Find a calm quiet space where you can gather your tapping script together using your negative belief statements and get ready to release the negative beliefs!

To begin, we identify the limiting beliefs that you hold about yourself.

For example, some of the beliefs that many bariatric patients have are:

I'll never be thin.

I'll always be fat.

I always sabotage myself.

I'm such a loser.

I'll never be successful.

It's so hard for me to resist food.

I have to have chocolate every day.

I crave chips (exchange chips for your food of choice).

Once you have a belief, or issue that you are struggling with, we will tap it out using the negative releasing statement by tapping through the tapping points.

Start with point 1 – (TH) top of head – using the statement below, then move on to the next tapping point 2 (EB) the eyebrow point, and so on.

Continue by tapping on the specific areas while saying the statement out loud to yourself.

EFT Tapping Points

1. (TH) Top of Head
2. (EB) Eyebrow
3. (SE) Side of Eye
4. (UE) Under Eye
5. (UN) Under Nose

6. (CH) Chin
7. (CB) Collarbone
8. (KC) Karate Chop
9. (UA) Under Arm
10. (IW) Inside Wrist

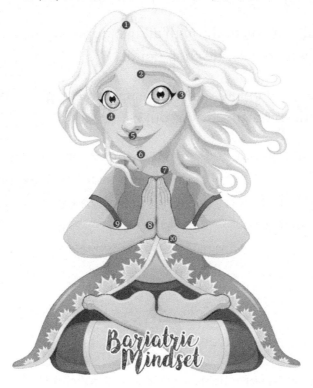

Tapping Scripts

Negative Release Set-up Statement:

Even though I (feel, believe, think) _enter core belief here_, I deeply and completely love, honor, and accept myself.

Repeat this statement through all the tapping points beginning with the karate chop point.

After you've completed the releasing of the negative belief, take a few deep breaths in and out.

Next, we'll use your new empowering belief to reinforce the positive statements to reprogram your subconscious mind. Please note that if you are still not in a place that you believe a statement such as:

I'm thin

or

I've lost all my weight and I'm keeping it off

Then start with something that is going to lead you down that road ... such as:

I'm open to being thin.

I'm open to losing all my weight and keeping it off.

I'm ready to learn what I need to learn to keep the weight off.

I'm ready to love myself fully.

I'm ready to lose all my weight.

I'm ready to release my trigger foods.

And so on.

Full positive belief statements are:

I love being thin.

Being thin makes my life easy.

I love my body and my body loves me.

I feel so good in my body.

It's so easy for me to resist chocolate.

My body loses weight easily.

These statements do not need a set-up statement because these beliefs are the ones we WANT to reinforce. The releasing statement is set up differently to let go of the OLD belief patterns.

This positive belief statement is always stated affirmatively and with positive words. Avoid using words like "not," "never," and other negative sounding words in your positive belief statements.

There are so many other statements you can create as well. These are just examples that you can use to begin your tapping routine. It's always better to find core beliefs that resonate with you. Each individual person will have different belief systems, so this list is not exhaustive of all the beliefs that could possibly be holding you back.

If you'd like to dig deeper into what you think may be holding you back, start writing things down that you think, feel, or believe about yourself. Then for the longer statements, make them more succinct or simplify them. This will help you create tapping statements to release the negative beliefs and install new empowering beliefs that will help you move forward.

MBSR (Mindfulness-Based Stress Reduction)

These exercises are less about food and more about de-stressing yourself and practicing active relaxation techniques.

For individuals who have trouble slowing down and being present, this is a great exercise to practice that. Starting small helps you to avoid boredom or a ton of mind-wandering.

These are easy, simple, and short. They help you focus your mind on the present moment, and through using your breath, this will also help you get more oxygen to your brain, which helps your higher-level thinking processes.

For many people who live in a state of anxiety, the brain and body are frequently in a state of fight or flight. Slowing down and breathing mindfully help you slow down and reduce autopilot behaviors as a result.

While these suggested exercises are very short, you can make them longer if you choose. Keeping them short gives your brain an opportunity to stretch and get used to being present for a short period.

Start with a lower time on the clock, and as you get better, increase the time gradually. 3–5 minutes is typically a good standard time; however, for beginners we'll start small and build from there.

❖ Exercise 1: 30 seconds of mindfulness

This exercise is about being in the present moment. Find a location where you can be alone for less than a minute. You can do this in your office, in your bed, or even outside.

My favorite example is during the autumn and taking a walk up or down the driveway. I will walk outside and listen for the sounds present. Intently listening I can hear the birds, the wind blowing, and maybe even a car coming down the street.

Then I listen even more, "crunch, crunch, crunch."

As my feet are moving, they are stepping on the leaves, which are creating the sound. Feel the leaves under your feet. Feel the ground under your feet.

What does it feel like?

What does it sound like?

What other sensations are you experiencing?

When you are using your senses, you are giving your attention to the present moment, and this helps you to relax and refocus your mind away from food and on the present moment.

❖ Exercise 2: 60 seconds of mindfulness

You can use additional examples other than the one above, and repeat this by increasing the time.

Some other examples are going for a walk, feeling the water in the shower, or even sipping on your water can be an experience in mindfulness.

Reflect on the moment and use three to five phrases to describe your feelings or observations from being "in the moment."

Shower example:

Close your eyes in the moment and get in touch with the experience.

The water is hot.

The water is pouring over my head and I can feel the water droplets as they hit my skin.

I can feel the heat of the water on my skin.

I can feel the steam as it hits my face.

I can taste the water as it enters my mouth.

Sipping water:

The water that touches my lips is very cold

I can feel the water drops as it goes past my tongue into my throat.

The water gets warmer as it passed my throat and goes down my esophagus.

❖ Exercise 3: Focus on your breath (30, 60, or 90 seconds, or longer)

This exercise helps you to focus your attention on your breathing and can help you lower your resting heart rate and blood pressure while you are doing it. When you do this, you are activating your parasympathetic nervous system, which signals your brain to turn down the activity in your sympathetic nervous system (the system that is stimulated during stress and activates fight/flight).

Additionally, when the parasympathetic nervous system is activated, it also promotes rest and relaxation while also triggering your digestion response. Your body is essentially calming itself down. This is also a great exercise in promoting a resting state such as sleep.

Take a deep breath in for a count of 4 ... 1, 2, 3, 4

Now hold it for 2 seconds and ...

Release your breath for 4 ... 4, 3, 2, 1

Repeat this 4-count breath exercise for 30, 60, or 90 seconds just being focused on your breathing, in and out ... in and out ... and so on.

Repeat this entire exercise as desired for tension release and stress reduction. Take note of how relaxed you feel after you've completed this exercise.

Progressive Muscle Relaxation

Progressive muscle relaxation (PMR) is a powerful relaxation exercise focusing on the muscles and different areas of the body to reduce stress and anxiety. This is a fabulous technique that when practiced regularly can help someone sustain relaxation for an extended period.

Additionally, it can help reduce stress and take you out of your head and into your body, literally by focusing your attention on your body.

The initial phase of this exercise is to focus on a specific muscle group, slowing tensing it, and then relaxing and releasing that specific muscle group. This exercise helps to focus the mind while also zeroing in on the specific muscle group and the different bodily sensations between the intentional muscle tension, and then the focused or intentional muscle relaxation.

Start near your head, beginning with the head and neck, then moving on to the shoulders.

Focus on this muscle group and tense them, then after a period of five seconds, release and focus your attention on relaxing this same muscle group.

Then move on to the next muscle group, such as your back muscles – tense muscles for 5 seconds, hold, then release and relax. Focus on the relaxation for a few seconds before moving on.

Then move on to your abdominal muscles – tense muscles for 5 seconds, hold, then release and relax. Focus on the relaxation for a few seconds before moving on.

Then move on to your hips/glutes (butt muscles) – tense muscles for 5 seconds, hold, then release and relax. Focus on the relaxation for a few seconds before moving on.

Then move on to your thighs – tense muscles for 5 seconds, hold, then release and relax. Focus on the relaxation for a few seconds before moving on.

Then move on to your calves – tense muscles for 5 seconds, hold, then release and relax. Focus on the relaxation for a few seconds before moving on.

Then move on to your toes – tense muscles for 5 seconds, hold, then release and relax. Focus on the relaxation for a few seconds before moving on.

Complete the exercise with a few deep breaths in and out.

Take note of how you feel after you've completed this exercise.

Visualization Exercises

As we discussed in chapter 3, visualizations help to reprogram your subconscious mind. What you see in your mind, you can achieve in reality.

We'll create a movie, the future you, just by visualizing your desired outcomes. You can do this as frequently as you like. Most of my clients report greater results when they are conducting visualizations multiple times a week. Also, they don't have to take a long time. Sure, you can sit there and visualize for 30 minutes, but, it's unnecessary. A few minutes a day, or 10 minutes a few times a week will suffice.

Take 10 minutes of time where you will not be disturbed or interrupted and move to a calm, quiet space. Allow yourself to be alone so you can focus your attention fully on your visualization.

Begin your visualization by closing your eyes. Take a deep breath in and center yourself.

Take a mental picture of the future you. What do you look like? What are you wearing? Are your clothes comfortable? How do you feel?

Experience your surroundings fully.

Where are you?

What's the environment?

Are you in a shopping mall, a forest, or are you on a cruise, or lying on the beach?

What do you see? Do you see a ship out at sea, or kids playing on a beach?

What sounds do you hear? Can you hear birds chirping or the sound of waves crashing on the shore?

Do you taste anything? The cool crisp taste of watermelon on your tongue, for example?

Do you feel anything? Like the wind on your face, or sand on your skin, for example?

Create the visualization by beginning to imagine the world around you. Use vivid colors and experience your world fully.

Use your imagination and get creative about where you want to see yourself.

Then put yourself into this mental picture. Repeat as desired for optimum results.

Take note after each visualization about how you felt. Also notice if your visualizations are helping you become clearer regarding your goals, or helping you reach your accomplishment faster.

This won't happen all at once, so don't get discouraged. If you plan to track how visualizations are helping you, you'll need to be consistent for at least 6–8 weeks using them a few times a week in conjunction with your other actions to help you see the greater impact on your mindset, and as a result, your behavioral changes that follow.

Journaling

Journaling is a great way to get inside your head. Another great way is to talk things out loud, so you can hear what you are saying and what you are thinking. The reason for both great ideas is that when you journal or get the information you are thinking/feeling out of your head, you can see it from a "filtered" perspective.

I'm sure everyone has had one of those "Did I just say that?" moments. This is why so many therapists, coaches, and psychological professionals tout journaling as a great idea. Inside your own head there is NO filter. When we discuss negative self-talk, you'll realize that the things you say to yourself are mean.

There are things you say to yourself that you just would not say to another person to their face.

Yet, you say them to yourself, "Did you see what you were wearing today, fat ass? I'm sure the office is completely laughing at you. What were you thinking?"

That's just one harsh example of what one of my clients wrote in her journal when she allowed herself to see what she was saying to herself on a regular basis.

Journaling has a great way of helping you get out of your head, so you can recognize what you are saying and NOT saying to yourself to help you better filter through the negativity.

Similarly, the self-talk can also sound something like, "Hey, let's just go through the drive-through! No one is going to know. You can just throw away the wrappers when you get home."

Again, the negotiation of the inner saboteur is loud and clear and there is no filter inside your head. But when you recognize through writing it down or talking it out, you can then do something about it.

One of my clients came to me and said, "If you are going to make me journal, I'm walking out! I hate journaling and it's not for me."

So that's when I got her to talk it out instead. I asked her to use her voice recorder or voice memo app on her phone to record her thoughts and feelings for ONLY her use. This allowed her to bypass the journaling, yet gave her the opportunity to get the same outstanding results of seeing what and how she was thinking in her deepest darkest moments.

I highly recommend journaling for those who want to dig into their own psyche regarding food and feelings behavior. However, if this is not for you, try using a voice memo or voice recorder so you can play it back to yourself and listen to your feelings. If you do decide to do this, see your thoughts/feelings with empathy and with different eyes.

Journaling Exercises

Take your time with each of these and try to write at least a page. I'm only sharing limited journaling exercises here as there are more journaling prompts scattered throughout this book that pertain to multiple areas of your journey.

What am I feeling today?

What have I noticed differently about my body today?

Am I excited or nervous about my journey after WLS? Why or why not?

What are my favorite foods so far after bariatric surgery?

What do you love most about your pouch?

What are you most excited about following WLS?

What are you most looking forward to after WLS, and why?

Keep a Success Journal & Focus on your Truths

Even if you hate journaling, a success journal is an easy way to help you track your progress. In your deepest darkest moments, your brain will conjure up all your past failures, how you are still a failure, why you suck, and all the hideous things you could say to yourself.

So, the success journal is more like a truth journal. You can write down things that happened, either actual milestones or things that happened on a day-to-day or week-to-week basis, which remind you that you are on track.

Example:

March 4th – Had a great day in the office. I was super productive, and I even avoided the doughnuts. Winning!

March 6th – Got on the scale. I'm down 3 lb.!! Woohoo!

March 7th – Had a great workout and my knees didn't hurt at all. How awesome is that?

March 9th – Finally fit into my size 16 jeans! Another size smaller!

March 10th – Dinner out with friends and I focused on protein first and felt satisfied pushing the plate away when I was done.

March 12th – Was tempted at a bridal shower today and I stuck to my plan. I committed to only having one bit of cake and that's exactly what I did!

March 13th – Decided to go for a 5-minute walk when I experienced some stress today. The old me would have gone for chocolate; I see how huge this is for me.

This is an example of practical steps you take daily or weekly or multiple times a week to take an inventory of activities that you are doing as evidence of your resolve. So, when you have a bad day, or a temptation, you can return to this journal and say to yourself "OK, I had a bad day, and look at all these days that I did amazing. I CAN do this."

The purpose of the success journal is to reinforce your positive behaviors, your successful behaviors, the times that you have overcome tough situations, to celebrate your wins, and to give yourself a shout out when you are rockin'.

This will help you focus on your accomplishments and realign your brain toward success instead of letting the negative thoughts step in, which can sabotage your efforts.

Food and Feelings: How to Recognize and Address Emotional Eating

For many, food can induce feelings of calm, comfort, and even joy. At holidays and big events there is always food. Food is associated with comfort and joy. Overeating, however, can cause serious health issues and when people eat emotionally over time, they are creating a conditioned response so that whenever an awkward or uncomfortable feeling arises, they reach for food.

Emotional eating is a habit. Just like brushing your teeth or brushing your hair, you may find yourself standing in front of the refrigerator asking yourself, "Hmm, what can I eat?"

By the time you've gotten there, you are likely looking for something to soothe you from boredom, anger, anxiety, frustration, tiredness, loneliness, or another emotion.

The first step to recognizing emotional eating is to track your patterns.

When and how often are you eating?

Is there a candy jar on your desk?

Do you fill it frequently or not often?

Do you reach into your desk drawer for a 3 PM Snickers bar?

What are your patterns?

If you don't know your patterns, it is time to get acquainted. This will help you grow.

Once you address what your patterns of eating are, you can begin to dig deeper into the emotional triggers that are popping up. Also, you can tell if it may be something else altogether. Being tired may not be an "emotional" state, but it is a physical state in which people look to food and fuel (such as caffeine) to get a "pick-me-up." Over time this creates a habit between your brain, your stomach, and your mouth.

"Oh, I'm tired, so this may mean I am also hungry."

From a behavioral perspective, we are conditioned over time when we do things over and over. So just like you can be trained to reach for a Snickers at 3 PM, you can also be trained to get up and go for a walk, or do some jumping jacks to get the blood flowing in your body, which is another way to wake yourself up.

Addressing emotional eating requires changing your conditioned behavioral state and doing something different. There is a saying, "What got you here, won't get you there."

Another great phrase is, "Don't expect to do the same thing over and over and get a different result." It's important that you engage new and healthy behaviors to help you build awareness that you are triggered to eat, and then deal with those emotions.

While the emotions still may come up, the way to change the habit is to first be aware of the emotional triggers, to take a step back when you experience them, and then consistently do something different over time. You will see over and over in this book, I'll talk about practicing awareness.

This is because when you're not practicing awareness, you are likely practicing habits, and habitual behaviors are autopilot "non-thinking" behaviors. The old patterns of behavior keep you stuck, and when you have a moment that you've "woken up" and realize where you are in your life, you become frustrated. This whole plan is about being conscious in your life and taking back control over automatic behaviors.

These are the steps to taking back control:

1.   Practice awareness of your behaviors (you'll hear me talk about being AWARE frequently).

2.   Look for emotional triggers that drive you to eat (why do I want to eat right now?).

3.   Shift your behavior when emotional triggers come up – meaning, do something differently (go for a walk, call a friend, journal it out, take a bath, get on social media, etc.).

4.   Feel the feelings fully. Yes, feel the emotionally uncomfortable feelings (this takes practice and patience with yourself).

5.   Name the feelings, or root of the feelings (I am anxious, tired, bored, etc.).

An example of this is to notice what your habit is, such as going through the drive-through at 4 PM.

Stop yourself and ask, "Is it time to eat?"

When the answer is no, ask yourself "What am I feeling right now?"

To go deeper, ask why you want to eat? You may see that you are bored, anxious, tired, frustrated, or any other number of emotions.

Examine your emotions, and if you can, write them down. This will help you keep a record of the emotions that are popping up. Then change the behavior by doing something differently.

Also, feeling the feelings fully is where some people get stuck because they may say, "Well, I don't know what I'm feeling."

So, if you don't know what you are feeling, begin by creating a mind map. A mind map is a series of words or thoughts that begin either in pictures or bubbles on a sheet of paper.

For example, you might get the feeling that you want to eat. You try to examine the feeling, but you don't know how to name it. Start small by going with the first thought or feeling that comes to mind. Name what you know and investigate for the rest. It will come to you, and this does take practice.

So many people avoid emotions because they are uncomfortable. Therefore, when you do begin to get to know your emotional patterns, it will be like a whole new world of YOU has been explored and exposed. This is awesome because you'll be able to shift your behavioral patterns and habits.

Start checking your physiological symptoms/reactions.

Is your body getting warmer?

Do you feel hot or cold?

Are you beginning to sweat?

Is your pulse racing, or is it normal?

For example:

I'm uncomfortable.

There is an uneasiness in my stomach.

I don't like this feeling.

Ugh, I just want to escape it.

What am I feeling?

My body is tense.

Am I anxious?

Am I fearful?

Am I scared?

Continue this process until you've examined the emotion that most resonates with you. This is another situation where you can pull out your voice recorder also instead of writing it down.

For many, there is something healing about talking it out loud. For others who may be more visual, using words or pictures will be more helpful. If you can't put your feelings into words, draw pictures. This can help you unravel the emotions, especially if you're good at pushing them down.

Allow them to bubble to the surface so you can explore them. Don't be afraid to feel your feelings. Getting in touch with them helps you to get to know yourself and your patterns better so you can overcome the negative behavioral patterns.

Once you can name your feelings, then you can work with them. Also, once you recognize your feelings, it will also be easier to identify the triggers as well.

Identifying Healthy Behaviors for Your Growth

Within the world of bariatrics, there is a topic discussed called "replacement behaviors." This topic usually comes up regarding a WLS patient replacing their food addiction, food issues, emotional eating, with another disordered behavior.

It's also referred to as "transfer addiction" from one disordered behavior to another disordered behavior. In other words, the WLS patient might take up drinking alcohol excessively, using/abusing drugs, excessive shopping, hoarding, sexual promiscuity, watching porn in excess, or the use/abuse of narcotics for pain management.

If this sounds like you or someone you know, it is important that they get into treatment or at the very least speak with their medical provider. Transfer addictions and replacement behaviors further hurt an individual's progress.

The root cause of their issues was not the food, but clearly, the food and weight gain were a by-product of something much deeper within them. It's highly recommended that they get in touch with an addiction specialist or look to engage in some type of addiction treatment. There are many resources available.

However, not everyone has this issue but still has issues with food, or may be seeking a form of neurological stimulation that they once got from food. Therefore, behavioral change is necessary and finding calming and self-soothing behaviors are necessary for long-term growth.

It's highly recommended that everyone has a list of at least 10–15 go-to activities that they can engage in instead of eating. This would help every individual who may be struggling with food triggers, emotional eating, or boredom so that they can "do something different" when they feel they need to cope with a situation and knowing that food is just not there for them anymore.

This is a great tool every WLS patient should have in his/her toolbox to maintain long-term weight loss and build healthy habits to deal with emotional stressors that do not include food.

Examples of doing something different, instead of eating:

Go for a walk.

Call a friend.

Write in your journal.

Take a bath.

It is recommended that you find your flow with some, any, of these exercises.

These exercises are for you to try. Get creative and try one for a period, or try them all sequentially. Feel free to use what resonates with you and ignore the ones that don't resonate. There will be exercises that excite you and others that you may not be interested in trying. This book is designed to help you pick and choose which exercises will be better for you as there is no one size fits all.

Chapter 7

Mastering Your Emotions

"Why can't I just say no to food?" she yelled, sobbing uncontrollably, "I feel completely out of control most of the time and I don't know what to do."

"I can't just expect my family to ban everything from my house, what is wrong with me?" she asked in a frustrated tone.

Kelly was 55 and had been married for 27 years. She was the matriarch of her family and while she loved this role, she struggled with trying to meet the needs of everyone around her, and as a result, she ate her feelings. She did not want to upset anyone, so she ate.

She struggled with her own feelings of insecurity and angst when someone else upset her, so she ate. When it came time to deal with confrontation, get-together's (celebratory or otherwise), she ate. In all situations, she shared, that her response to her feelings was eating.

We didn't discover this on day one of our work together, but when we did discover it, it was a big aha moment for her. For many of the clients I work with, food and feelings become comingled. In our world, food is something that we have traditionally throughout most of all the things we do.

Whether you are attending a wedding, baby shower, funeral, or graduation party, I promise you there will be some kind of food present. Eating is what we do best as a culture, and as a result, we have a huge issue with obesity. Food has become more than nutritional nourishment for our bodies, it has become a socially acceptable activity having nothing to do with actual physical hunger.

What bariatric surgery does is, it reconnects the patient with actual physical hunger. As you go through the essential elements for bariatric success, there are certain nutrition requirements: protein, water, eating more fibrous vegetables, lowering one's carbohydrate intake, using vitamin supplements, not drinking when eating, moving your body, and so on.

However, you will still be subject to social situations and food. You will still experience emotional triggers to food whether they are stress/anxiety, anger, happiness, or boredom. The feelings will pop up and if you haven't dealt with them, then now is a good time to begin.

The truth about food and your feelings is that this whole process is not about the food at all.

Surprise!

You might be thinking, wait, wait, this whole process is about eating and food.

Yet it is not!

Yes, the food is important and what you are choosing to eat is important; however, the reasons behind the choices are what is really driving your behavior.

The pleasure centers of your brain say, "Ew, protein oatmeal! No, thanks!" And then they scream loudly, "I really want a burger and fries!"

The point of having bariatric surgery is threefold: to lose weight, move with ease, and to enjoy life.

Getting to this successfully requires that you change how you talk to yourself and that you change your habits. We've talked in-depth about behavioral changes and long-term habit shifts, and now it's time to discuss how you talk to yourself.

How do you speak to yourself? Think about that for a second. Let it sink in.

What's the self-talk like inside your head?

The truth is, we don't have an internal filter when we talk to ourselves, and so most of the time, the self-talk is very harsh.

Just like you wouldn't tell your best friend," Hey, fatty, it's time to hit the gym," why would you say that to yourself?

You would most likely say to your friend, "Let's go to the gym," instead of talking her out of it.

Friends offer support, they value you, they call you out on your own BS, and they stand up for you. This is what you want to go on inside your own head. Instead, you may have the inner saboteur offering you Ben & Jerry's after a long day rather than encouraging you to go for a walk.

Other times, we rationalize, compromise, or give in to things because it's more difficult to stay accountable to oneself because of the inner saboteur.

The dialogue inside your head goes something like this:

Self: UH, what a long day, I'm so tired! Yes, and there's no dinner. Hmm, I can just pick it up. OK, protein first.

Saboteur: Wait, but I really want that chimichanga. OMG! That would be delicious.

Strong self: Self, you can't have that. It won't fit. It's too much food ... and there's not really a lot of protein in there.

Saboteur: Well, we'll carve it up and eat the protein first, of course.

Strong self: What about the shell?? Won't that be too many carbs?

Saboteur: Oh, come on, you'll only have two bites!! Come on ... we are hungry, just order already!

Strong self: Maybe I'll just get the grilled chicken.

Saboteur: Really? It's not like you go out often. Just get the chimichanga, you know you love the cheese dip inside!

Strong self: It's really not a good idea. Oh God, I'm so hungry! I need to just order.

Saboteur: This is a one-time thing, just c'mon and order it already.

Weakened self: OK, just this time, I mean, I don't really eat that much, which is true. I'll just get that. I can be good next time.

Do you see what is going on here?

Rationalization. Manipulation. Minimizing the issues. And, so inside one's own head, the saboteur typically wins out.

This is what has caused the bigger overarching problem in the first place!!

Learning how to shift your mindset and master your emotions is integral to your success in the long term because you can be your own best friend or your own worst enemy.

There is an old Native American parable that I usually share with my clients:

An old Cherokee chief was teaching his grandson about life ...

"A fight is going on inside me," he said to the boy.

"It is a terrible fight, and it is between two wolves."

"One is evil – he is anger, envy, sorrow, regret, greed, arrogance, self-pity, guilt, resentment, inferiority, lies, false pride, superiority, self-doubt, and ego."

"The other is good – he is joy, peace, love, hope, serenity, humility, kindness, benevolence, empathy, generosity, truth, compassion, and faith."

"This same fight is going on inside you – and inside every other person, too."

The grandson thought about it for a minute and then asked his grandfather,

"Which wolf will win?"

The old chief simply replied,

"The one you feed."

– Author unknown

This is an important parable to share because each of us has an opportunity to feed the "good wolf" or the one that will carry us to success. However, the negative voices exist. The sabotaging self exists. The deeper the emotional wounds of the past, the more important it is to encourage the positive and denounce the negative.

This doesn't mean the negative voices will completely dissipate; however, when you focus on which voice you want to grow, you'll begin to see changes occur within you, and as a result, in your behaviors as well.

Likewise, it's important to realize that no one is positive all the time. There will be times when you'll experience anger, rage, greed, resentment, and so on. However, when you have the tools to deal with those emotions, and when you express them in a healthy manner, they will not stay bottled up inside you.

Having outlets to deal with these emotions is important so that you do not turn to food to deal with your emotions.

History, Causes & the Theory of Eating Behaviors

Looking back to how we got here as a society, it's been creeping up over time. The society we live in is very fast-paced requiring quick eats with little preparation, so we can devote time to other things that we deem more important. When it comes to the way that modern life has changed us, it is important to realize that the ideas of eating too much and working out are new.

In the past, our ancestors were focused on working as little as possible since most of the work was in the field to grow crops or hunt for food. It was also very important for those who were eating to eat as much as possible. When you think about the idea of slight obesity, you remember that it was a sign of wealth in the past because it meant that the person was not obliged to work in the field. Now, however, it is very clear that while these were the ways of the past, now it is necessary for people to work out and to not overconsume.

It's important to note that the food consumed by our ancestors was not processed like it is today. Processed foods can cause digestive issues in some people because that's not how nature intended for us to eat. The point is, the desire is still there within our biological makeup, and subconsciously we don't discriminate between processed or unprocessed foods. The brain may be hardwired to tell us to conserve energy as well as to eat more.

It is important to be aware of what you are eating and why. From an emotional perspective, there may be a need to eat beyond the physical and beyond the biological, and for many people, the emotional urges are satisfied with comfort food. Also from the past, food has long been a tradition bringing family and friends together. Therefore, today when celebrations happen, people eat. When there are sad events like funerals, people eat. For just about anything and everything, as a society, people eat.

Getting off the Emotional Eating Rollercoaster

When you shift your mindset away from eating as a coping mechanism or to calm down, and look to eating for actual nourishment, things begin to shift. Practicing awareness is key.

Even thinking the question, "What does my body need?" helps you to ponder this.

Does your body *NEED* chips, Cheetos, Oreos, or M&Ms? Absolutely not.

Yet, these are foods that more people eat daily rather than occasionally because our culture has because a candy/cookie food culture focused on pleasure eating, and eating for filling an emotional need, rather than one focused on nutrition.

Just like you would not run your car on gas that would cause it to die before it hit 100,000 miles, why would you feed yourself food that could shorten your lifespan?

Yet, as a culture and society, we do it every day. The logic in this is simple, yet we are socially and culturally programmed to eat this way because it is acceptable and pleasurable. This is where the shift needs to occur for you to get healthy for the long term. The healthy foods that sustain your body nutritionally need to be at the forefront of your diet rather than the processed foods.

Likewise, it's important to evaluate what comes up for you emotionally when you think about cutting those things out of your eating plan. This helps you look at the excuses and to realize that they are just that.

Your brain might come up with ways that you "need" ice cream or cookies (or another trigger food) in your life for one reason or another. You may come up with more ways why you still "need" soda.

However, I guarantee, if you go to any doctor with any issue, they will likely tell you the exact same thing that I'm sharing here, that you do not need soda, or cookies, or crackers, or ice cream to live, and in fact those items eaten in pre-surgery quantities are most likely harming you more than helping, even if you think they make you "feel better" emotionally.

The emotional hit that you get from a sugar high is due to the changes in your brain chemistry. There are scientific articles that discuss the issues with sugar and other processed foods in our society. However, is the short-term emotional satisfaction worth the long-term pain?

Most people say yes because we live in a very instant gratification society.

Additionally, because you may have made it a habit of eating these types of foods on a regular basis, it has become the norm. Then, as a result, you experience unhealthy results, weight gain, and other health issues.

Yet, when asked to give them up or to change your patterns of behavior, you may get extremely self-protective, self-justifying, or defensive because change is uncomfortable.

The good news is that this process of shifting your mindset happens one step at a time, and while it will stretch you, you'll build new healthier patterns that help you feel better inside and out. This is also why mindset work is so important.

Temptation is everywhere, and the goal is not to increase your willpower but to change your mindset around food, starting with utilizing strategy.

It's not about getting you to say "NO" to ice cream 100% of the time per se, but instead asking yourself, "How can I eat something enjoyable that will also sustain my body?"

The purpose is to refocus your attention on the consciousness of eating rather than responding to your emotional states with food.

This way you avoid the excuses that you give yourself when faced with the temptation of a trigger food. When evaluating the options, this helps you strategize and come up with a different option instead of returning to your old pattern of eating foods that don't nourish your body.

Likewise, mastering your mindset is all about managing your emotions. Excuses pop up when you are presented with trigger foods: "I'll just have one," or "I'll work out later, I'm so tired." These are part of the old behavioral patterns.

Taking a stand for yourself to do something different is a change you need to make daily to get where you want to go. Each person has a "WHY" or a deeper reason that they've had surgery.

For me, I did not want to die. I did not want to end up like my parents stuck inside their house asking for help because they were so obese they could barely move to get around without feeling very exhausted. I saw their struggles, and I did not want to live that life.

My deeper "WHY" has to do with living a life that is full of life rather than full of TV. It's about playing with my son, watching him grow up by attending his activities. I knew that if I didn't act, I would be couch-bound, and again, that's not how I want to live my life.

You are here for similar reasons. Your WHY is huge for you. You have something to live for. What is it?

Is it time that you take a bigger stand for your life and get off the emotional eating roller-coaster?

Let's begin.

Digging Deeper, Slowing Down, & Being Conscious

You already know how fast-paced our world is. I don't have to give you statistics or share how we sometimes work 12–15 hours a day, look for quick meals, quick fixes, and prefer 15-minute anything to deep, dark boredom. The truth is, most of us are doing anything and everything we can to avoid two things: boredom and digging deep within our emotional selves.

Emotions!?!? Ick!

Who wants to deal with that?

In fact, it sounds like such a downer. Of course, people avoid it, because what typically comes up when you dig into emotional work???

One word.

PAIN.

So, just out of curiosity, who likes to deep dive into a free-for-all in the self-induced pain archives??

Anyone?

Anyone?

I thought so.

While some people are really excited about digging deeper into their emotional consciousness, there are even more people who avoid it.

Enter food and other coping mechanisms.

Please note that while not everyone who has bariatric surgery is a food addict, most are emotional eaters. It's also important to share that even individuals who are not obese or have not had bariatric surgery, can have issues with eating emotionally.

Getting in touch with yourself and building awareness is the first step in changing the behaviors. When you are aware, you're able to check in and then doing something different.

Doing something different is about checking in with what matters most to you. This slowing down and reflecting help you to make conscious decisions. Another point to make here is emotional eating versus conscious decision-making.

Some people can say NO to foods when the emotions are removed and replaced with a conscious decision. For emotional eaters, the emotional high that they obtain from food is calming; therefore, that's what they reach for.

However, when using a tool to slow themselves down and regain perspective, they also regain control over themselves, and as a result, the food and their eating behaviors.

My client Bree had weight loss surgery three years before we began working together and shared that she struggled with emotional eating. Her goal was she wanted to be able to push food away confidently and with ease. She shared that some days she would struggle with stress eating due to her busy and overwhelming career as an event planner, especially when a lot of her meals were provided for her as part of her job.

She would typically be on location at the event side all day and so would usually just eat what they provided. We worked on her mindset around food, not focusing on what she had to give up, but instead we focused on the decisions she was making for her present and future self.

Every time she went to a party or event, which was frequent because of her role, I asked her to check in with her consciousness to use four criteria. I asked her to check in with herself emotionally and to ask herself if a specific food was right for her to be eating at that time, if the food was something she wanted at that moment, if it was something that would nourish her body, and if she felt an emotional pull rather than a conscious choice.

Using this strategy became a huge success for her because she as she used it more frequently, she became aware of her patterns, and as a result, was able to say NO more frequently.

At her first wedding event, after beginning to use this strategy, the bride really wanted to give her a piece of cake. Bree said that she checked in with herself and although she was mentally/emotionally tempted, she recognized after doing the check-in that she really didn't want it, it would not be nourishing for her body and politely turned it down. She told me later this made her feel powerful and could hardly believe she turned down cake.

Her second event was a funeral/wake event that she planned for over 500 people. She told me she was very stressed, and that there was a lot of finger food everywhere including cupcakes. She shared that the cupcakes triggered her. She really wanted to eat them in addition to some pigs in a blanket she noticed on another platter, which she said she hadn't had in years.

Then, she said that when she checked in with herself on this occasion, she was drawn to these foods mainly because of their emotional appeal to help her to soothe, not because she "really" wanted them. She said it would have been fulfilling an emotional void, not because she was drawn for any other reason. She also counted this is a huge win because she knew this was a tough situation where she was both hungry and stressed and that this was a double whammy for her.

At a third event, she attended another wedding that she had been the event planner and coordinator on. She shared that she was looking forward to this wedding very much because she had worked previous events for this family, and they always took care of her well. She also had been invited on this occasion to have a piece of cake by the bride in addition to having been provided with a plated dinner, which was normal for these types of events.

At this occasion, she said she accepted the cake and sectioned off about two bites of cake that she could eat and felt satisfied. I asked her what was different about this event, and how she felt about it. She shared that this time, it wasn't about the emotional need and that she felt it was a conscious decision made because of checking in with herself.

She shared that she felt both satisfied with her decision and felt no guilt as a result. This had been a huge mental shift for her because previously, she would have said yes, no matter what, and this was a very conscious "yes" that was not grounded in fear of hurting someone's feelings, or an emotional need to eat, or an emotional desire arising from stress.

Although Bree had used this strategy at times previously and had unsuccessful attempts, I share these three specific very successful attempts here to highlight the practice of stepping back and looking at your choices.

Additionally, Bree knew this would not be a skill or strategy that would transform her overnight. We worked on this for a while helping her to tackle the inner saboteur and the voices that had once held her hostage. Bree's awareness of herself and her needs helped her create a foundation that she can draw from and feel confident in when making food choices, which has changed her eating behaviors.

Reflecting and checking in with yourself is important because this helps you to see whether you are reacting or responding to food.

In my own experience as a WLS patient, I too have had urges and episodes where I just wanted to eat even when not physically hungry and when not at a mealtime. In fact, one of my biggest goals was to be able to feel good, proud even, about my food choices and to push food away and feel so amazing on the inside.

The old me would eat and feel icky and self-loathing. I hope that these tools that I've used myself and with my clients can help others also say "no," more frequently, with greater ease over time, and exceedingly with greater confidence and pride in their decisions.

How Do I Measure Something I Cannot Name and Always Avoid?

The process of identifying your emotions does not need to be an arduous one. You just need to be consistent.

It is likely that you have the same feelings and emotions come up over and over, and over again. It is likely that you avoid the negative emotions completely while allowing yourself to experience the more positive ones on a lukewarm level.

Just like you may avoid the negative emotions, being so happy, or too overjoyed throws you off too. This all goes back to the deeper beliefs of being unworthy, or not deserving of really awesome experiences and things. So, you tend to avoid feeling TOO good, just like you avoid feeling TOO awful.

Feeling too much is just hazardous, so it's avoided.

So, when you can't feel it, you definitely can't name it. So, how do you change it?

The practice of feeling your feelings is an exercise for the person who is READY to do the deep work to heal their emotional wounds.

It takes you back to your past, through the muck, the gunk, and all the stuff that caused the pain to begin with. While there are strategies and tools to help you get a hold of your emotional eating and practicing the awareness, the sifting through feelings and naming them, this is where the real mindset work begins.

Start with a feelings chart. Have this handy chart close by when you want to know what you are feeling, see appendix B.

Then look at the list. What feelings or emotion closely resonates with what you are feeling?

Write it down.

Then ask yourself: Am I done? Is this it? Or, is there more?

You may find that you have more emotions than you realize that are ready to come out. Remember that once you've identified your emotions clearly and regularly, you can begin to act on soothing them without food.

If you get stuck after identifying the emotions, please remember you have all the tools in this book to move through them. If you become overwhelmed with emotion, use one of the tools in chapter 6 or in this chapter to help you move through those emotions so that you can break through your emotional barrier. Remember, this is your opportunity to do something different rather than the old habit of turning to food.

It may be uncomfortable at first, but I promise it will be worth it once you work through the feelings and get to the other side.

If you feel this is too deep to do on your own, please reach out to a therapist or counselor to work through these exercises.

E3 – Exercise, Excuses, and Your Emotions

Kicking your excuses to the curb is essential. The first step to doing this is naming them. What excuses do you carry around that keep you in old behavioral patterns?

Once you name them, then you can make sure that it is possible to take back control and bust through them.

Excuses are everywhere when it comes to working out because it pushes you outside your comfort zone. Regardless of whether it is cold, or you are tired, there is no reason for you not to get in a good workout. Whether or not you go to the gym, you can get a good workout in anywhere.

A part of the success or failure of your journey is that you need to make sure that you are going to see the excuses when they are happening and to act so that you are going to find a way around them. This is the mindset piece. If you've been overweight or obese for a while, it hurts to work out. I remember the days when my knees and feet would take a pounding, and of course when you experience pain, there is a message that goes to your brain, the one that says, "Stop doing that, it hurts!"

This is where you need positive reinforcement instead of negative reinforcement. The pain is negatively reinforcing the exercise, meaning that you are reinforcing the "let's not do that again" feeling. However, if you feel awesome after a workout, that's positive reinforcement for your brain. This is why the mindset piece is so important.

Many times, you may think that there is a situation that allows for an exception; however, with further inspection you may see that it is an excuse. Then once you allow an exception, it's easier to give yourself permission over and over again, causing this to become a habit.

Habits don't just pop up. They are built over time. An example is when someone brings doughnuts in on Friday and puts them in the break room in your office. Your first thought is either damn them or hell yeah, doughnuts! That shows where you are in your thought process.

When you decide that is not on your plan and you stay consistent with that, when that happens, you have certainty without a doubt that you will not have a doughnut. However, if you must wrestle with yourself each and every week, whether you will succumb to the devouring the doughnut, you have not developed a habit of saying "no." Instead, you have to have the internal fight.

"Doughnut or no doughnut, that is the question."

This leads to mental and emotional anguish because of sitting on the fence decision-making. What I mean by that is, when you don't decide, you mentally walk by the break room one hundred times, "Do I or don't I?"

Then you make a pros and cons list inside your head, and then you rationalize what you could eat later that would save calories, or maybe you could skip lunch.

Then you justify why you should have the doughnut, and this mental self-talk can go on for hours. To save yourself the headache and many lost work hours, decide and release the "maybe." In the long term when you say "no" to the doughnut, you are also building the neuropathways in your brain to help you say no again and again and again.

This becomes your new normal, without a doubt, on the regular. Sure, you'll be tempted, but you'll more often stand firm because you know what is important to you in the long term, and we'll talk more about this in goal setting.

But, when you say "yes," then you've opened that door mentally and emotionally. Then the next time you have doughnuts in the break room, it gets harder and harder because the neuropathways in your brain that you have reinforced have been the ones that are "doughnut-friendly," and the next time the doughnuts arrive your brain will seek out the doughnuts for the sugar high it provides, and it will be more difficult to say no.

However, you may also be well informed that you are using this as an excuse and that the food is not something that you really need and still do it, anyway. This is the emotional piece surfacing to fulfill a nonfood desire using food.

In other words, you are using food as a coping mechanism to deal with stress, uncomfortable situations, anxiety, or any other range of situations. The point is that if this is common for you, you are probably using food to cope with life issues instead of dealing with them head-on.

Compassion ≠ Permission or Self-Indulgence

When I look back at my own eating behaviors, it was easy for me to comfort myself with food. The smell, the taste, the experience of eating was exhilarating. At the same time, I felt shame because I was obese. This forged a big conflict because socially, it is unacceptable to be fat, yet, eating felt so good. However, the pattern that I continued for quite some time was one that I thought mostly resembled compassion.

I was hurt, so I ate.

I was happy, so I ate.

I was sad, so I ate.

I was frustrated, so I ate.

Do you see the pattern? Do you relate to this pattern?

The realization that I came to was that compassion was the same thing as permission, and now I know it is not. We've all seen the movie scenes where the lead character breaks up with her boyfriend and goes and eats a pint of ice cream. This is what we are shown in the media as normal behavior, and as a result, we normalize it in our own lives.

Similarly, in my own life, if I was down, sad, happy, struggling, frustrated, angry, fill in the blank with any emotion here _____, as a result, I ate. Emotional eating is a very large issue; however, to focus here is about the difference in compassion versus permission (to eat) or the act self-indulgence because they are, in fact, not synonymous.

It was after attending a conference a few years ago and studying the work of Dr. Kristin Neff, that I realized how important self-compassion is for individuals healing from their struggle with obesity. In Dr. Neff's work, she discusses how self-compassion is important for individuals to understand because it is part of the human experience, and knowing how to comfort oneself when suffering is essential.

What is Self-Compassion?

According to Dr. Kristin Neff, self-compassion is "extending compassion to oneself in instances of perceived inadequacy, failure, or general suffering" (Neff, n.d.). She also has defined self-compassion as being comprised of three main components: self-kindness, common humanity, and mindfulness (Neff, 2003).

What is Permission?

Permission in this context is allowing yourself to engage in a behavior that conforms to your habits, norms, or makes you feel comfortable in the moment. Example: you may give yourself permission to have a doughnut on a Friday.

This is also not the same as compassion because the idea that it is permissive to have a doughnut and if guilty feelings follow, it adds to feelings of inadequacy rather than relieving them.

What is Self-Indulgence?

Self-indulgence is the "excessive or unrestrained gratification of one's own appetites, desires, or whims" as defined by the *Merriam-Webster Dictionary*. This is much different from self-compassion because it means that an individual is engaging in self-gratification over self-love or self-kindness. It's clear they are not the same.

Using this as a guide, become aware of how often in the past you may have used food as kindness, or have been permissive with food to feed your feelings. These are both permission and self-indulgence rather than self-compassion.

Self-compassion comes from a place of self-love and understanding the difference and practicing the application of the differences can make a huge difference in your life. You'll start loving yourself more, and in turn feel more confident in your relationship with food.

The Controversial Topic of Self-Love

As a bariatric patient myself, I remember prior to surgery all the talk and hype about self-love, self-love, blah, blah, blah.

I didn't understand it, and in fact, I thought all those people who told me that "I just needed to love myself more" were a bunch of fruit loops.

I mean, seriously? Love myself?

Come on!

Then came weight loss surgery, and the influx of emotions that I'd been avoiding, very much like my clients.

I had to deal with them because the food was no longer there. Well, it wouldn't be there if I wanted to lose the weight.

So, as I dug into my emotional dungeon, I realized for myself, that my whole relationship with food, eating, and the emotional roller coaster had a lot to do with the self-loathing that existed within me. Although I've always been bubbly and extroverted, the pain of inadequacy, worthlessness, undeserving, and "not-enoughness" was lying there beneath the surface, waiting to seize me as I tried to take on the goal of really knowing myself.

The realization that self-love was something I avoided hit me like a ton of bricks.

If I ventured into that territory and actually began down that path, I'd have to feel the feelings, which we all tend to avoid; and then, I'd have to do the work.

In my work with my clients, I help them dig deep to see what exactly they are struggling with, within themselves. Not everyone has self-love issues, and I've had many clients who openly share and state, "I completely love myself."

Be clear, this is not an issue for the whole population. However, it is one that is highly avoided and can be very controversial because of other areas in therapy where people think that self-love fixes everything. It does not.

Self-love is just one aspect of the bigger picture. Just like eating to soothe your emotions is just one aspect of a bigger picture.

Each are parts or segments that help understand the complexities of human suffering and human needs.

We all need something different, and from childhood we may have missed out on love, or somehow it may have been modeled that we weren't worthy, deserving, lovable, and so on.

The act of self-love can help open up many doors and help ease emotional eating by allowing you to see clearer who you are and who you are meant to become.

Be aware of it and be inquisitive. Is this an area where you struggle too?

Do you love yourself, or do you just think you do?

Even if you think you are confident and secure in who you are, think about your behaviors and whether you act out of fear or love for yourself?

Reflect on this and write notes in your journal.

The path to self-love is similar to the path of getting to know the new you. It takes time, and awareness is the first step.

❖ Self-Love Exercise

Start by writing down things you LOVE about yourself.

Begin with physical characteristics.

Then write down personality characteristics you love about yourself.

What awesome things are you best known for?

What makes you most proud of you?

What do you love most about yourself?

Reflect on your answers and check in with the insight this gives you about you.

❖ Conquering Your Self-Talk

We all know that what you say inside your head makes a difference for your mindset. This is why it's important to tie all of this together. Your self-talk is instrumental to your mindset work. If your headspace is negative, you may get stuck frequently, whereas when you know how to encourage and empower yourself, you can shift your mindset more quickly.

❖ Self-Reflection Activity:

Make a list of all the reasons that you want to be healthy. You will see that when you do that, you can plan to reassure yourself with positive reasons why you want to pay greater attention to your health. This also helps you take a look at your self-talk.

Positive Self-Talk: This ensures that you are going to move forward with self-control as well as make great change. This type of talk is encouraging and supportive.

Negative Self-Talk: This will lead you down the path to excuses and to failing at the path you are on because it is typically self-critical, harsh, uncompromising, and hateful.

If your internal dialogue is one of encouragement as well as one of self-control that will allow you to continue with success. If you are in a situation where you are shopping for food, you have to make sure that you are not bringing food into the house that is not on the list that you can have.

You may think you are depriving your family of some foods and other items they may want. However, you will see that it is very important to make sure that you are not filling your house with things that are not going to be on your list.

"I can't change the direction of the wind, but I can adjust my sails to always reach my destination." – Jimmy Dean

At the end of your day, reflect on what you may have said to yourself. It's impossible to evaluate all your self-talk, so just reflect on it in hindsight.

Is it kind? Is it mean?

Write down some keywords, phrases, or statements that you say to yourself frequently.

Do these statements reflect how you feel about yourself?

What do you say most often to yourself?

Are they kind? Are they mean?

❖ Learning How to Talk to Yourself

Listen to Your Dialogue: You want to make sure that you are listening to the way that you are talking to yourself. Are you setting yourself up for success? Are you making excuses for your situation? Are you being positive or negative?

Have Personal Catch Phrases: You may find yourself wanting food and also being tempted. Make sure you have come up with a list of phrases that are just for you that will allow you to be able to ensure you are going to stop yourself when you are tempted.

Talk to Yourself When Stressed: When you are stressed you may find that your go-to is to return again to food. You want to make sure that you do not do this. You need instead to focus on being proactive and stop yourself when you are in that moment. Use phrases you have developed that work and get rid of the ones that do not work for you.

Confront Your Anxiety & Do Something Different: When you are in a situation where you used to eat when you felt anxious and you are not eating, you will see that you are going to have more anxiety. It is important to find something else and new to do with that energy. Go for a walk, call a friend, or attend a support group meeting. If you have a therapist, make an appointment and go. Engage in a hobby or join a club.

Deep Breathing is Your Friend: If you find yourself in the situation where you are having issues and you need to pause, plan on having a deep breathing technique. Try to allow yourself to breathe for about 30–40 seconds and you will feel better.

Stop Yourself: When you are in the moment of having a panic attack or when your anxiety is increasing, you need to imagine a stop sign in your mind. This is a great way to pause yourself and ensure that you are able to have a moment to collect your thoughts.

Remind Yourself WHY: When you are in a situation that you feel like you need to eat something, ask yourself what happens if you don't. You will see that in that moment the desire to eat is strong, but it is more important to focus on the long-term goals of your health and your wellness.

Additionally, this is a good time to whip out your journal and write about what you REALLY desire at this point. The short-term gain of the food is not worth the long-term struggle you'll experience with regard to trusting yourself around food.

Journal It Out: Write out your feelings, even if they are harsh, and reflect on them. Write to yourself as though you were writing to your best friend, husband, or wife. What would you say to someone you love who really needs to change their own self-talk? How would you encourage someone who you know needs to be lifted up? Take note of this and reflect on it.

❖ Turn Your Negativity into Positivity

You need to remember that when you are in the moment of having negativity, you need to turn it around with these techniques quickly. This is your mindset shift. There are many reasons that you may want to return to your prior habits and situation but you need to see that that moment of weakness can take you off course.

Everyone struggles with this, but just like building muscles, we've got to build your mindset as well. The old way of thinking may have been, "Well, why not have the ice cream, what will it hurt?" and subsequently giving into the food. The new mindset is about standing up for yourself, your goals, all that you have achieved so far, and reminding you how far you've come.

The path of shifting from negativity to positivity is not about being airy-fairy or fluffy, and in fact, it's about getting real with yourself and your behaviors. Start by naming things that you know for a fact you are good at, and what you've already accomplished. Use truths to help you shift out of a negative mindset, into a more positive one using facts of your past to empower you that you can do it again.

❖ Emotional Shifting Exercise

Be aware of your goals and state them in a positive manner.

Know when you are making an excuse or falling back into old patterns.

Stop yourself in the moment and reframe the situation (Is this going to help me or hurt me?).

Push yourself through excuses.

Ask yourself, "What have I done before that has been successful?"

Take action in the present moment.

Celebrate your successes.

Remember Your Visualizations: Your Photo Album for the Future

Make sure that you create a photo album of things you want to do in the future, and maybe a way you want to look. Then get an image from this book in your mind when you are tempted to cheat or eat off-plan.

At the end of the day, what you decide to do or not do is going to lead to your success or your failure. You need to always ask yourself if you are bringing yourself more toward success or failure with the decisions you are making.

Decisions are huge because when you decide something you are in your conscious mind. When on autopilot, you are acting on a habit, not a decision. Therefore, this is a great tool to use to help you make a conscious decision in the moment, and not leave it to habit or that old autopilot thinking.

Additionally, this brings you back to your big WHY. Your big WHY is the reason you had surgery to begin with and when you are in that conscious state, you'll practice the habit of the new mindset, which in turn leads you to the new behavior.

"Every great dream begins with a dreamer. Always remember, you have within you the strength, the patience, and the passion to reach for the stars to change the world." – Harriet Tubman

❖ DO-ing versus BE-ing

DO-ing versus BE-ing is an amazing self-awareness exercise you can do just about anywhere. It begins by taking inventory of your behaviors.

What exactly are you doing?

Who exactly are you being?

Are you BE-ing the old you, or the new you?

Are you DO-ing things the old you would do or the new you would do?

So many of my clients are DO-ing the work. They DO, DO, DO. They are following their plan and doing their exercises; however, they have not yet grasped the idea of BE-ing the new person they planned to BE-come after bariatric surgery.

There is DO-ing. Then, there is BE-ing.

Who you are BE-ing has a lot to do with what you are DO-ing; however, the two are not always comingperforled.

My client Michael was BE-ing the person he wanted to when it came to his food, but was not DO-ing the work he needed to at the gym. He resisted. When he hit a stall, he complained. Then he started DO-ing the work at the gym, and he started gaining muscle and losing fat. He realized how his lack of DO-ing, contributed to his stall and weight loss resistance.

For example, my client Ava had not yet stepped into her confident self and she hit a stall. Once she released the emotional baggage from her BE-ing, the physical weight was easier to lose. She had finally begun to assimilate to the person she was BE-coming.

Here's another example. Marcy had lost 98 lb., which was a huge win. However, she was still wearing her baggy clothes that did not fit her. She had no problem affording new clothes, but she wasn't used to being so small. Marcy was DO-ing all she needed to do the work for herself and her body; however, she had yet to step into the BE-ingness of the new person she had become.

She felt an emotional blockage, and when she shifted out her wardrobe, she began to attract new people into her life, and even gained a promotion. Once she BE-came emotionally who she was ready to BE, other things shifted in her life.

❖ **BE/DO Exercise**

Write down the tasks are you DO-ing to become the new you?

What is it like to BE the new you?

Are you stuck in either the areas of BE-ing versus DO-ing?

Take an inventory of your responses and use these to gain insight into your behaviors.

❖ **Following the plan**

No matter what, following your plan will be one of the best things you ever do. Over time you'll be tempted to shift off your bariatric eating plan. Whatever you do, stick to your plan. These guidelines will help you stay on track and keep you successful. For your emotional health and well as your mental health, the plan was created to help you lose long term, and keep it off.

Sometimes there is more emotional stuff comes after regaining, so ensure that you are on track so that you don't enter the path of regain, and keep the weight off for life!

Chapter 8

Relationships after WLS/Bariatric Surgery

Not all relationships are created equal. You'll have people who support your decision to have surgery and those who don't. You'll have people who you tell and people you don't tell. Your bariatric journey is your own, and it's important that you go through this process having people in your life who support you, love you, and are there to cheer you on as you succeed.

Of course, there will be people who are jealous, struggling to understand your decision, or have a hard time with all the changes you are making in your life. This is about them, not about you. However, they will make you think it's about you.

Friendships: Dealing with Jealousy, Anger, and Other Issues

Maybe for a long time you were the token "fat" friend among your group, or maybe you all have been obese together. When this is the case in either situation, unless you have friends who are extremely supportive and encouraging of your weight loss, there can be some people who don't know how to handle your weight loss.

You may even have friends who suggest you both "get an appetizer" when you go out to dinner after surgery just like old times. They may be happy for you, but, they miss their OLD bestie, and they want you to stay the same. While at first sight, this may feel like sabotage coming from your BFF, it may just be that they miss that old part of you, and they don't know how to interact with the new you. Therefore, vulnerable conversations are so important with those who are closest to you.

It's important that you ask your friends for what you need and remind them that you are the same person. Your confidence will rise, and at times, you may not feel like the same person, and they might not feel you are the same person, yet at your very core, you are the same you and you'll want your friends to cheer you on! Of course, who wouldn't?

This is a time when all relationships, even friendships are put to the test.

Take my client Melanie as an example. Melanie was 28 and single when she had weight loss surgery. She and her best friend Amy were both obese. Melanie was ready for surgery, but Amy was not. Amy was very supportive at first, she was excited for Melanie's decision and started to think about surgery for herself.

After Melanie had surgery, she had spent quite a bit of time recuperating and wasn't as engaged as a friend, this hurt Melanie's feelings especially after all she had been through. She eventually reached out to Amy, and Amy admitted she didn't want things to change between them and expected they would.

Having an open and honest conversation about your feelings, and about your expectations of the friendship, can help you both save the relationship, or at least, help you both come to an agreement. More anger and resentment occur when there is distance, uncertainty, and when people turn their backs to one another.

Isn't this surgery about me? Yes, and no. It is about you, and yet your friends and family will think it is about them too.

The thing is when you have surgery, people can be happy for you, scared for you, and even when this is all happening in YOUR life, they are thinking about how it will affect them.

Within human psychology, people are typically thinking about "Well, how will this affect me?"

No one says this out loud, and most often, people don't even realize this is how their reactions and responses develop. So, the next time someone says something to you, or about you, ask yourself, is this about me or is this about them? Give that some thought and reflect on it.

What could they be missing out on because of your surgery?

What issues could pop up for them if you change who you are?

Maybe they fear you'll find a new best friend and leave them in the shadows.

Maybe they fear that once you lose the weight, you'll feel "too good" to hang out with them anymore.

The important thing to remember is that many of these emotions that come up that cause them to be insensitive or resistant to your decision to have surgery, is about them, not about you.

This is also a time to determine whether you want to maintain friendships with those who are not ready to accept the new you, or have trouble with staying the course of their own sabotaging behaviors.

Listen to your heart and do your best to reach out and ask your friends boldly and blatantly what they think. If they choose to not support you, it is their loss.

Romantic Relationships

Are you married, in a relationship, or single?

What does your relationship history look like?

Take a good look at who you were allowing into your life, who is in your life, and who you want to be in your life from this moment forward?

❖ **For the singles**

Dating after WLS is a topic I'm asked about frequently. It is not that different from dating prior to WLS, except that you are much thinner, and you are perceived differently. The question I ask many of my clients is how they perceive themselves in the dating process. This is because many individuals may still have that "obese thinking" that integrates low self-esteem with "not good enough," and when you throw in boundary issues, it can be a huge mess.

As an amazing individual, you have great things to offer in a relationship. However, the negative cyclical thinking that you may have to "settle" or accept the first person who gives you attention may pull you back into the same old pattern of relationships that you engaged in prior to WLS, and we both know that's not what you want.

The surgery changes your physical state, and as a result, you feel differently about yourself. However, the mindset portion of this requires that you change yourself, and your behavioral patterns, so that you can raise your standards to meet a partner worthy of dating you, loving you, and being in a relationship with you.

At 367 lb., I was single and looking for love. Even now, after 7 years of marriage, I remember what dating felt like.

I remember posting skinny-fat pictures of myself, you know, just the head and shoulders and hoping that when we met in person that they would ignore the thick thighs wedged in some Spanx. I'd hoped that the Spanx would hold in enough fat that I would pass as slightly overweight, instead of morbidly obese.

Who was I kidding?

Everyone wants and needs love. This is part of life. Finding quality relationships is difficult when you deny any love for yourself. I always knew I would get married and have kids. It was just something that I knew wholeheartedly without a doubt.

However, my weight had generally fluctuated between 345–375 lb., and I wasn't sure how I was going to meet the partner of my dreams. My self-esteem and self-worth were at an all-time low because of how I saw myself on the outside. Clearly, I know now that my inner reality was reflected in my outward appearance and not the reverse.

Sometimes, however, it feels like a chicken and the egg type situation. The outer reality also affects the inner dialogue that sounds something like this: *Look at you, who would want you?*

My dating history had been plagued with bad boys, love 'ems and leave 'ems, one date wonders, and then that one long relationship that broke my heart into pieces and left me feeling that I was not worth loving.

Doesn't everyone have one of those?

In my journey of self-awareness and in my private practice, I realized that many obese women, like me, struggle with self-doubt, self-esteem, self-trust, boundary setting, and really struggling with believing that they are good enough to find a partner.

In my experience, I had a relationship that focused entirely on my weight. Of course, now I see that this breakup was the best thing that ever happened to me, but at the time, it tortured me, because it reinforced my "not-enoughness." It was the relationship that ended because, in so many words, I was just "too fat to love," and he'd marry me if I had just lost the weight.

I hid this for a long time because although I wanted to find love, I wasn't sure if I could because the weight seemed like the biggest thing in my way. As a result, I attracted people into my life who treated me as badly as I felt about myself, which then just perpetuated the cycle.

This book is not all about love and relationships, yet I have to bring these things into the awareness because when someone struggles with obesity, it affects so many other things like their self-worth and self-esteem and it is reflected in their behaviors.

As I grew, I saw the patterns of behavior that I held which were incongruent with who I wanted to become, and I had to change that if I were to change into the person I want to become. I knew I had to hold myself to a higher standard in order to attract people who were of a higher caliber, and as a result, I did.

In contrast, however, I would then do things to prove my worth in other areas of my life. I went and got an advanced degree. I would take on more than I could handle so I could validate myself as "good enough." I tried to show people that I was "worthy," when deep down inside, I was struggling to find myself worthy of anything. Some people might see this as depression, while I saw this as a cry for help.

I looked at how I was denying myself greatness. Instead of settling for whoever would give me attention, I started to write out a list for the kind of person I wanted to attract into my life. This is an exercise that I share with my clients as well. I like to call it the "main squeeze" exercise. In this exercise, you've got to upgrade your mindset and start thinking about who you want in your life and how they'll add value to your life and in a relationship.

Likewise, think about the value you bring to a relationship. This will help you see that you are lovable and worthy.

Do this exercise to get clear on who you want to attract in your life, and the type of person you are looking for.

❖ **Are you ready to date after WLS?**

Main Squeeze Exercise:

Start to brainstorm your ideal partner.

As a single, make a list of the characteristics you desire in a partner. Do NOT compromise. Do NOT settle.

If you want something, go after it.

Make a list of personality characteristics you desire in a partner.

Make a list of physical characteristics you desire.

What are your non-negotiables?

I always tell my clients to list non-negotiables – things you MUST have, because these are things you would not settle for, ever.

Does he/she need to be college-educated?

Should he/she hold a job? Have a car? Live on their own?

Also, make a list of things that are deal-breakers. Deal-breakers are things that rule this person out as a potential partner. This will help you get super clear on the type of person you're seeking.

For the Already Married WLS Patient: How to Maintain or Improve Your Marriage

If you are married, stop and look at how your relationship looked before weight loss surgery.

How did you treat each other?

What ongoing issues did you have with each other, if any?

Have the two of you had any discussions about the changes that the weight loss might bring about in your relationship?

Have you discussed the need for additional emotional support?

Have you discussed what changes it would bring to your household eating habits?

These are some great topic discussions to bring to the table with your spouse so both of you are on the same page and can help support each other regardless of who is having the weight loss surgery.

When you communicate your needs, it becomes easier to discuss with each other and to ask for what you need. Likewise, your partner will find it easy to ask what he/she may need from the marriage as well. Remember, this is a two-way street, where both of you get to discuss your needs and desires for the relationship, as the goal is to grow together through this process.

Who you were before bariatric surgery and who you are after may be very similar, or you may become drastically different. This depends on you and the changes that occur within you along the way. It also depends on the types of relationships you had prior to your surgery, the type of person you were before, the type of person you are in a relationship with, and how much you've grown after your surgery.

My client Sarah had surgery in 2012 and was married prior to surgery. She was ecstatic to get the surgery and like many of us, saw it as an opportunity for her to FINALLY lose the weight and feel great about herself. Her husband, however, was very jealous and feared losing Sarah as a result of her physical change.

Sarah's confidence had soared following surgery, and this also helped her to change jobs and even go back to school to pursue an advanced degree. As a result of all of these changes, her husband's behavior became radically abusive and overly controlling.

He'd require Sarah to check in multiple times a day with who she was with and even had her enable a tracking app on her phone, so he could locate her at any time. Jack, her husband, refused to go to marriage counseling and insisted that Sarah's surgery had ruined their marriage.

Additionally, Sarah felt that Jack would try to sabotage her weight loss success by purposefully buying snack foods not on her plan to get her to eat them and regain weight. Unfortunately for both Sarah and Jack, they divorced in 2014. I met Sarah in 2015 following her divorce from Jack and struggling with a period of regain because of the emotional turmoil.

Sarah shared with me that she didn't understand why Jack was so needy, and was frustrated by his attempts to sabotage her. In the end, she realized he had somehow won as she struggled with 35 lb. of regain, which she was working hard to reverse and pick up the pieces of her life simultaneously.

Not all relationships are this difficult; however, this gives an idea of how important relationships become and how instrumental partners can be in terms of weight loss or in weight regain.

Maryell's story is a little different.

Maryell was married for 10 years prior to having bariatric surgery and her husband was very supportive of her having a gastric bypass. He helped her removed the processed foods from the cabinets, would assist her with meal planning, and helped her stay on track.

Allen, Maryell's husband, cheered her on as she lost weight and neared her goal. Allen would go walking with Maryell, and as a result, they got fit together. Allen had never really had a weight problem, but his blood pressure was out of control. Through supporting one another, they got healthier together, and so did their marriage.

One of the biggest changes that occurred between Maryell and Allen was their communication and understanding of what they both needed from the marriage, from each other, and they discussed how they could support each other in the process. Maryell didn't know what to expect, and neither did Allen. However, because they prioritized their health and communication with each other, they succeeded together.

Each relationship is different, which is why it is important to begin communicating early in the process. One of the biggest things that can help a couple in this process is communication and seeking to understand the other person's point of view.

If Sarah and Jack had sat down, and discussed the changes as they were happening, and had Jack been open to discussing his feelings, they might have been able to save their marriage. Clearly, Jack was unable to be vulnerable enough about his feelings with Sarah and was so afraid of losing her that he did everything he could to sabotage her success.

Of course, this is not what we think of as love, and this is clearly an example of how some relationships are simply not healthy. This is also a good reason why some couples really do need to reach out to a marriage or relationship counselor following bariatric surgery to gain a greater understanding of the emotional and physical changes that are happening, so they can continue to grow together and build on their marriage.

There are several other reasons why marriages may struggle or fall apart after bariatric surgery; however, it's important that if marital issues appear on the horizon that you ask your partner to open the lines of communication, so you can discuss it together.

Going through weight loss can be a challenging process for relationships. Arguments can ensue, miscommunication is rampant, and people can get super frustrated. This is when the individual requires even more compassion for their partner, not less. Weight loss is a process and for many, it can be viewed as a big sacrifice, when, in fact, many people gain so much more in life as they lose the weight.

Five Ways People Can Navigate Relationships through the Ins and Outs of Life after Bariatric Surgery

1. Try to see things from your partner's perspective

The weight loss process can be short and sweet or long and tedious. Although there is so much more to gain in terms of weight loss such as increased movement, healthier body and mind, and improved overall wellness, some people get lost in "why" they are on a plan because they can get frustrated with the process. Try to see things from the perspective of the person on a weight loss plan.

Your partner may have gotten on the scale and realized they gained weight, and now they are frustrated.

This is not the time to say, "I told you so!"

This is a time to be more compassionate and to address the behavior in a kind and loving way. This is also a time to see things from their perspective. There could be a lot of shame and guilt that has built up, and rubbing their face in eating behaviors will not help them to grow, instead, it will likely drive them back to eating because of the stress and overwhelm from a negative conversation. This is not healthy either. Asking your partner to discuss their feelings is important and seeing things from their perspective might shed new light on the situation.

Likewise, if you've seen your partner work hard, and they are struggling, try to see how you can offer additional avenues of support.

Where can you lend to the situation?

Can you help watch the kids so they can work out?

Can you put the kids to bed, so your partner can get to bed early?

What energy are they putting into this?

How might they be feeling during this time?

Looking at it from a different perspective helps you to see that it might not be all sunshine and roses and that they are working hard to lose the weight.

2. Be kind to each other and communicate effectively

As you are changing your diet and exercising, your mood can shift quickly. This can sometimes leave little patience or lead to frustration in general. Therefore, it is important to be patient, kind, and understanding of the weight loss process. For one person it may seem clear or easy, and for another person, it may seem like climbing up a hill with ten-ton bricks on one's back.

Within relationships, we rely on clear communication to understand one another, and for healthy relationships to flourish. When someone's mood is off, they can be snappy, short, or curt. Some call this "hangry," which is a combination of hungry and angry.

The food-mood connection becomes very clear here. When going through a weight loss some people can feel deprived, and as a result, overly moody. Revisit #1 to see things from your partner's perspective.

Say what you mean and mean what you say, always trying to be sensitive to your partner's feelings. Listen to what they have to say and really digest it. Also look for ways to be kind yet straightforward. Sometimes when people sugarcoat things, it can be misinterpreted.

Asking for clarification or confirmation of understanding can help.

Can you clarify what you just said?

Did you understand what I meant?

Men and women communicate very differently, and so it's important to clarify and ask questions when in doubt.

3. BE THERE ... Ask how you can help & give emotional support.

Ask. Ask. Ask. Then ask some more about how you can help. This is a journey. Your partner will likely welcome the emotional support, as well as support in the kitchen with cooking healthier meals, and maybe even as a workout buddy.

Not all couples will work out together and that's OK. If you do things together though, it can help the success rate. If you are someone who wants to help your partner succeed, be there for them, but be careful not to be a nag. Nobody likes the food police, or someone hounding them about getting to the gym. Support is good, just be sure you're not overdoing it.

If your partner doesn't want the direct hands-on support of assisting with dinner or going to work out together, also be understanding of that too. Instead, ask how you might support them indirectly. It might just be that you need to be a listening ear on the more difficult days. Remember this is a process and there will be ups and downs.

4. Give encouragement

For each, and every person, it's important that they are encouraged and recognized for the work they are putting in on their weight loss process.

Encouragement helps people to feel they are not alone, and especially in a relationship, it helps when recognized by one's spouse/partner. This also builds intimacy as it helps the other person realize that his/her partner is paying attention and is participating in the process, even if on the sidelines.

5. Be considerate

Once a client told me that her husband wanted to help her celebrate her 50-lb. weight loss by taking her out to dinner. While she appreciated his kind gesture, she recognized he hadn't realized that by celebrating with food, it could potentially sabotage her weight loss.

They discussed it and he confessed he had not even thought about it that way, shared that he was excited for the dinner for himself, and he had not been dealing with weight nor did he have a weight problem.

Therefore, being considerate and thoughtful of the other person's journey is important. Also, it's important to look at your own intentions when going out to eat.

Is your partner avoiding chocolate cake?

Is that a trigger food?

Then why take him/her to a cake shop?

Things like this help avoid disaster and support the relationship through thoughtfulness.

Celebrate Success with Your Partner

Losing weight and feeling great should be celebrated, so why not do something together or share some kind words of celebration to show your partner you care. As noted above, going out to eat is not the best choice for a celebration; however, you can do many other things that do not include food to celebrate one's weight loss success.

It can be through words of encouragement, flowers, love notes, or doing something like going on a hike or taking a trip or tour somewhere together.

"YAY!"

"Way to go!"

"I'm so proud of you!"

"I knew you could do it!"

Words and support go a long way. Let them know that you've noticed and you're there for them no matter what. That's what helps people grow together: leaning on each other and supporting one another through it all.

Overall, there can be a lot of benefits from partners losing weight together or in general. It helps boost mood and overall health/wellness. This helps partners do more together and get around easier. Being a supportive and considerate partner during and after the process also helps support long-term weight loss.

Setting Healthy Boundaries

Are you a "Yes" person?

One of my favorite sayings is, "What you allow, is what will continue."

This phrase is very poignant when it comes to having healthy relationships and boundary setting. You want something to change, but you don't know how to change it. You fear standing up for yourself because you don't know what the other side of that looks like. However, when you allow the behavior or situation to continue, it will.

Long before weight loss surgery, it is likely that you were saying "yes" to people about things you would have much rather said "no" to. However, you didn't quite know how to say "no." This is much more common than you may think.

The truth is, "No" is a complete sentence.

Many individuals have a subconscious need for approval because they feel bad they are unable to do or manage things due to the excessive weight, or they are trying to overcompensate for other reasons.

My client Angie had trouble saying "no" to her boss because she felt if she took on more work, that she'd gain a promotion.

After digging a little deeper, she shared that she felt she needed to "do more" because she was the biggest person in the office and she had overheard one of her coworkers refer to her as a "lazy ass." This left Angie feeling like she had to pick up the pace to gain favor with her boss, her department, and at work.

Likewise, my client Greg believed that if he helped more at his church, he'd gain additional recognition. However, at home, his wife complained that he was never there, and as a result, their marriage suffered. Greg was addicted to the external approval because he received more praise, whereas at home, he was expected to do chores and duties, and was rarely recognized when he did things in the home.

He said "yes" to doing more at church and "no" to doing things at home, and as a result, he was praised at church and ridiculed at home. He struggled with maintaining any kind of boundaries because he would not let anyone know how he was feeling, and as a result, ate more to soothe his discomfort.

In other situations, there are WLS patients who cannot say "NO" out of guilt. I've seen this pattern frequently with my clients who feel bad that they can't spend time with friends and family like they wish they could because they just cannot move. So, they say "yes" to other things that they would otherwise say "no" to, just to avoid confrontation, arguments, or to gain approval, or to feel better when feeling bad that they are unable to commit in a more active way.

Therefore, saying "yes" is what they do out of convenience, to gain acceptance, or out of obligation or to avoid being called out on their own weight issue. There is an underlying fear of being rejected due to a combination of excess weight and low self-esteem.

This often becomes a pattern or habit and even after weight loss, if nothing changes, the pattern can stay the same unless the individual decides to do something differently.

This can take shape in many forms.

- ✓ It can take the shape of taking on extra work at one's job to gain approval from the boss or manager.

- ✓ It can take the shape of always saying yes to your clients, rearranging your schedule, or running around finishing something.

- ✓ It can take the shape of not standing up for oneself in an abusive relationship. Allowing people to treat you poorly even when you know it's not right, fearing they won't love you if you do say something.

- ✓ It can take the shape of letting people walk all over you.

- ✓ Ignoring a cheating spouse out of fear he/she will leave you.

- ✓ Helping someone even to your own detriment (losing excessive amounts of money or time).

- ✓ Giving things to others to keep them around or to earn love/affection/attention.

Setting boundaries is scary, especially when there is fear that you would lose your relationship, job, partner, friend, and so on.

The truth is, setting boundaries and standing up for yourself helps you to gain the respect of those individuals, and by standing up for yourself, they will respect you more. Will they like it at first? Probably not.

However, when you start to shift and set healthy boundaries regarding what you can do, are willing to do, you actually gain the respect of those individuals and they know where you stand.

A few months back, one of my clients came in with precisely this issue. She had recently had weight loss surgery and was used to overcompensating in her role for taking on a lot of work. She shared that she was exhausted, but that she felt she had to take on the extra workload to prove her worth, and that she felt threatened because of her weight.

After she had surgery and at a point when she had lost about 60 lb., she shared that she was ready to "do her best" in her role, but was not willing to take all the extra work she had used to do because she felt taken advantage of.

She feared she would be let go, seen as lazy, or that people would notice her doing less and would be "at risk" of losing her position as a result. She specifically feared having a talk with her boss about doing a "normal" workload without all the extra hours.

She feared this because she was not used to setting boundaries and because although she was well on her way to losing weight, she still thought she wasn't worthy enough to set such boundaries.

In her words, she asked me, "What if they think I'm just not good enough doing just my normal job?"

It took some time, but she finally spoke to her boss and told her boss she would be focusing on herself more, and while she would complete all of her normal duties, and while she's "glad to help in a pinch," she wouldn't be regularly taking on extra workload like she had for the past several years.

To her surprise, her boss replied, "Well, it's about time you focus on you, you deserve it!"

My client was dumbfounded and also elated. Her fear was that she would be looked down on, and the truth is, the only person who was looking down on her, was herself.

Many individuals who have struggled with obesity see themselves as pariahs as outcasts, and as a result, try to "do more" or "be more" for others almost apologetically for their weight. This is how poor boundary setting becomes an issue and honestly, a horrible habit.

It's out of self-loathing that people try to gain love, acceptance, approval, and in the end, it just ends up hurting them more.

While I strongly believe this has got to stop, it starts by shifting the self-hatred to self-love. It also begins by setting better boundaries and believing you are worthy of healthy relationships/friendships, healthy work settings, healthy homes, and so on.

It is also understood that people who set healthier boundaries live more fulfilling lives. Having good boundaries in relationships and at work is linked with lower stress levels, increased life, career, and family satisfaction.

Isn't it time that you started saying "NO" to what doesn't serve you, and "YES" to what will?

Here are a few steps toward setting healthy boundaries.

1. Evaluate your current situation.

In what area(s) of your life do you believe you have let boundaries slip? Is someone taking advantage of you consciously, or are you allowing yourself to be used, or utilized to your own detriment? Are you being pushed around or manipulated?

In what area or situation in your life would you like to say "no," yet time after time, keep saying "yes" to people, situations, or things that aren't serving you?

Write these down so you can look at them clearly. There may be more than one, and it's OK. You'll take each, one step at a time.

It's important to evaluate what you're saying "yes" to and what you're saying "no" to. Are these situations ones that you can change, or not? Would better boundary setting help your situation?

Being clear about this will help you in the next steps.

2. What are your fears about setting boundaries in this situation? Write them out.

Writing out your fears helps to get them out of your head. Most people have fears that they never play out on paper, and they seem worse than they are. That's why this step is so important.

You may fear that the person or situation will spiral out of control. You may fear losing someone's love, attention, or affection. You may fear losing your job, shifts, respect, your clients, and so on. You may fear that someone will get more manipulative and threaten you if you stand up for yourself. You may fear that by standing up for yourself, you'll lose more than you'll gain.

Write this all out, get all the stories out of your head to help you evaluate if there is any truth to this, or just fears you've created in your mind.

3. Set small steps: What small steps can you take to start setting healthy boundaries?

Just as you looked at your fears above, by looking at the "small steps," you can begin to see that you'll do this over time and not all at once. Too much all at once is overwhelming, scary, and likely to keep you stuck in your old ways. By setting boundaries one small step at a time, you'll begin to taste the victory, see the respect shifting, and will likely do it more and more.

Another reason to shift slowly, in setting boundaries, is so that you don't upset the apple cart too much. This could also harm relationships. If suddenly, you go from a softy to rock hard in your delivery or demeanor, the people who are used to thinking you are a pushover will start to push back as well.

Let's say you're like my client who took on too much work.

Let's say she just said, "You know what, I'm not doing this anymore. I've done this for years, and no more!"

The response would probably have been completely different. She still offered to help when the company needed her, but she set a boundary that she wouldn't be doing the extra work while sacrificing her own health, free time, and so on.

It's important that the right communication is used and that small steps help ease others into the new boundary-setting you, so that they don't think you are angry, resentful, or completely changing too quickly.

If you change too fast, people can push back on your efforts and make you feel guilty for setting boundaries to begin with.

Another client of mine had a husband who she caught cheating multiple times. Before she had weight loss surgery, she shared that she just "dealt with it" and frequently felt shamed about it, but after surgery, she wanted to see something change.

She started by having a conversation with him about their relationship and his behaviors and what she knew all along. As you can imagine, this wasn't an easy conversation; however, it was much easier than her yelling, screaming, and/or giving him an ultimatum.

In the end, she ended up seeking a divorce; however, he knew it was coming especially since she had set the boundary that she was no longer going to put up with a husband with a straying eye.

Looking at what small steps you can take, even if it is just a conversation, are good things to think about so that you can start taking action sooner rather than later.

4. What is likely to happen when you start to set these healthy boundaries? Write it out.

As noted above, if you act too fast, people are not going to like it. They might accuse you of changing, thinking you are "too good" for them, or that you are "too good" to work hard, or even that they liked the "old you" better.

Most people don't like change, this is why acting slow and steady gets them used to the changes, and gets you used to making these changes.

Just like the old saying, "Rome wasn't built in a day," neither are personal boundaries.

It took you years to get to where you are, so why do you think you can flip a switch and change everyone's reactions to you? This will take time, but stay the course and start back at step 1 when you get confused.

What do you really want to change?

Who keeps pushing your boundaries, and why does it make you uncomfortable?

What would you like to see differently?

Know and be ready for someone to challenge your new boundaries. Be prepared to stand your ground, because if you don't hold your new boundaries, you've taken two steps back.

If you cave after they push back on your boundaries, then they really won't respect you and you'll be teaching them that they can push you around. Or, you'll be sending the message that you weren't serious to begin with, which will further hurt your future attempts at boundary setting because they will push back even harder.

However, when you stand firm to your new boundary, people are more likely to respect you and honor your decisions, whatever they may be. They may not like it, but they WILL honor it.

It's time you start to ask for what you really want, recognizing that others may not at first like the "new" you, but they will respect you when you put yourself first, and when you honor your boundaries, others will do.

5. Take action. (Set that boundary!)

It's action time. It's time to start setting your new boundaries, no matter how scary it may seem.

The more practice you get, the easier it will become, and you'll wonder why you didn't do this sooner.

You may need a little more bravery to each step and that's OK. This is why you start small.

Taking action can be both exhilarating and scary at the same time. At first, you may experience fear not knowing what the reaction will be, but once you do, you'll start to set more boundaries after you see that people do respect you and the decisions you make for yourself in your life.

Sex and Sexual Advances after WLS

Sex may a touchy topic to discuss; however, it's a very necessary topic to discuss for WLS patients.

Most of my married clients share that WLS has made their sex lives more fulfilling and enjoyable. Many of my single clients have differing takes on this because there can be emotional issues that arise after WLS concerning sex or their sexuality, specifically some have feelings that they are only lovable or sexually desired as a thin person and this can affect their mindset. This is an important issue to unravel as the whole person is deserving and worthy, not just the new thin self.

Some of the WLS patients who I've come across in clinical practice have endured childhood trauma or sexual abuse in their lives, which may have led to them overeating to ward off future potential attackers. While some WLS patients welcome sexual attention after bariatric surgery, others are terrified of it.

Sex in general after bariatric surgery can be very satisfying due to the loss of excess weight, increased endurance, and ability to gain closer proximity to one's partner.

For those who may have had sexual issues in the past, or have a history of trauma, it may be a good idea to work with a therapist on these specific issues. Sometimes, people gain weight to insulate themselves or appear unattractive to possible predators. This is a way that individuals attempt to stay safe if they have been victimized in the past.

Survivors of sexual abuse may need additional counseling or therapy because there may be issues that come up in your post-op weight loss surgery process where the inner saboteur is loud.

Although the weight loss saboteur may be the same saboteur that is trying to keep you safe from harm, it would be important to work through these issues with a professional trauma specialist so that you can be successful.

For many individuals who have not received many sexual advances prior to surgery, there can be an increase in your sexual prowess and attractiveness following your extreme weight loss.

It's important that you establish a mindset that gives you some insight into yourself and your own sexuality as well. Here are some good questions to reflect on and ask yourself after surgery.

How do you feel about yourself sexually? What potential sexual issues do you foresee?

Do you notice any sexual changes?

Do you have any fears about engaging in sexual activity?

Do you have any fears about people finding you sexually attractive?

What other thoughts/feelings arise regarding sex or your sexuality because of bariatric surgery?

Chapter 9

Staying on Track and Avoiding Regain

"Fall down seven times, get up eight." – Confucius

There will be times in your life that you struggle to stay on track. There will be times that you may even want to throw your hands in the air and say, "I give up."

I hope that the tools and techniques outlined in this chapter and in the rest of this book guide you to stay on track no matter what. Everyone has a bad day occasionally, but getting off track for a long-term period is much more about an "oops" than it is a total derailment.

Essentially, it's a return to old bad habits and usually has something to do with the inner saboteur that tries to return full force to say, "I told you so."

The negativity in this process has to do with fear, sadness, struggle, frustration, and typically an uphill battle with yourself.

There will be tips that come up in this chapter that may seem like they repeat from other places within the text. This is on purpose because I've decided to put them here as they are related to staying on track and avoiding regain.

They are more than "eat on-plan," and "practice your routine," or "remember to exercise," and more psychological in nature. In previous chapters, the basics are clear.

In this chapter, we're going to go deeper into why regain happens and how to practice self-awareness, so you can avoid the pitfalls and stay on track.

Staying on track has to do with many aspects of emotions and behavior. It also has to do with dealing with difficult life stressors and issues you don't expect and yet need to deal with.

Regain always occurs as a result of, "going off the plan." There is no other way to put it. When more food goes in, and less activity occurs, you are headed for regain. This does not mean you have to exercise more.

Instead, this means that no matter what is going on AROUND you, you still need to be CONSCIOUS of what's going on WITHIN you.

There are several reasons that people "get off track" or "go off their plan." Life stressors are a major reason because they are the leading cause of emotional instability. While people may have a diagnosis of depression or anxiety, these are likely to decrease after surgery.

While others might be susceptible to depression after surgery due to a loss of their sense of self, self-identity issues, or a lack of clarity of who they really are, others may gain a renewed sense of purpose. Following surgery, there is a big probing question that emerges, "Who am I now?" This pops up for many people, while others may adjust easily.

Any of these issues could lead to regain if not addressed. Food is an outlet that some people turn to when they don't want to deal with uncomfortable situations. Digging into deep questions like, "Who am I now?" can be stressful and overwhelming. When it comes to life stressors, it is most likely that distress or negative life stressors would be a more likely cause of weight regain than eustress, or positive life stressors.

Examples of Distress are:

Divorce

Death/loss of a spouse or family member

Miscarriage/stillbirth

Loss of a job

Loss of a home

Life-threatening illness or health diagnosis

Examples of Eustress are:

Marriage

Birth

Home purchase

Promotion

Cross-country move

Graduation

Changing jobs

Big life issues can trigger old habits to come back into play. It's important to stay vigilant with the basics and reacclimate oneself to the bariatric basics during a time of high stress.

Going back to the basics is essential for getting back on track or staying on track after weight loss surgery. The BASICS are a necessary element of post-bariatric surgery success. If you feel you've fallen off the wagon and are approaching regain, or are already there, use a meal planner, journal, and/or food tracker to help you stay accountable. Get an accountability partner or buddy to help you stay on track.

If you feel you are having serious emotional or mental health issues, then it is strongly recommended that you reach out to a counselor or therapist to get additional support.

There are short-term and long-term effects as a result of dealing with positive and negative stressors.

The short-term psychological and physiological responses are to plan for such events, because these are typically events you can plan for.

The long-term psychological responses are depression, anxiety, long-term stress, getting out of your normal routine, and possibly a return to old autopilot habits if you're not careful.

This year (2017), I lost my dad. It was the end of February. We spent the whole week in the hospital, he passed the first week of March. I had a lot going on and remember how efficiently I ran everything because I had my own emergency plan in place. Loss is never convenient, and typically very emotionally overwhelming. You never know when it will happen and then, it just does.

What helped me to stay on track was having many of the tools in this book at my fingertips. I had my non-negotiables list, and I knew what foods I could eat, and which foods were an absolute NO.

I knew that I could walk around the hospital to get my exercise in, and I conquered the urge to emotionally eat by staying busy and surrounded by family.

Everyone will need to develop his/her own process for this just as I did for myself, and as I do in session with my clients. Having plans, for when life takes a left turn, will help you stay on track.

I've met many people who have had to care for a sick parent or child and the overwhelm is so great that they forget to take care of themselves and regain the weight.

Remember that you are important and that your weight loss is to not only help you but also affects those around you. Your life is important, treat it as such by caring for yourself enough to prepare in advance.

There are situations where people do not want to feel the emotions of a crisis situation, especially if they have been doing so well at avoiding their feelings for this long. Feeling the feelings can be difficult for people and this can be another source of regain, not getting in touch with oneself or digging deep into the mindset work.

Doing the necessary mindset work helps people stay on track in the long run and helps them become prepared for when obstacles appear, and life throws you a curveball.

Effects of Emergency Mode

Reactions vs Responses / Emotional State of Overwhelm / Working on Autopilot

Reactions are instantaneous and typically driven by beliefs. This is when the unconscious mind is running the show. Responses are thought out and given more cognitive consideration, which are driven by the conscious mind.

Reactive behaviors are not always the best because they don't involve the decision-making process. When you program your mind to respond, through shifting your mindset around food, you'll be more in charge through your conscious mind, than your unconscious or subconscious mind.

When in a state of overwhelm, you can get into a very reactive state driven by autopilot behaviors. Your brain doesn't know what to do first when it is overloaded.

Create a priority list and follow it. Keep it brief and simple. This will help you to stay on task for what you need to get done.

When autopilot is revisited, and old habits are reengaged, weight gain usually occurs. I cannot stress enough the importance of utilizing your new tools to keep you on track.

Create your meal plans, write your grocery list, and stick to your plan. Make this a non-negotiable, no matter what.

❖ Have a Crisis Management Plan

Even when you think everything is planned, nothing is planned.

No one knows when a crisis will hit. When you have a plan of action for that, you'll be better prepared. Even having a week's worth of easy meal plans in the bag can help you stay the course when you may be working 15-hour days, shuffling the kids here or there, and might even be making hospital visits.

Make a list of healthy fast foods so that you are not tempted to order something overly fatter or heavy on the carbs.

When in doubt ask yourself: is this pouch-worthy?

Also, create an easy exercise routine such as chair exercises or a simple walking routine that will help you stay fitness-focused no matter what is going on around you.

New habits can go out the window quickly when crisis strikes. Even when nothing is planned, have a backup plan to help you stay organized. This will help you stay in charge of your life and your WLS journey even when the unexpected occurs.

❖ Recommit to Yourself and Your Process

No matter what is going on around you, the most important thing is what is happening within you. When you notice yourself getting off track, it's time to recommit to yourself and the process.

Small steps forward create leaps and bounds over time. As Darren Hardy discusses in his book *The Compound Effect*, it's not what you do one day that really matters, but what you do every day that counts. The effects of your behavior add up over time, and it is essential that you pull yourself back on track as soon as possible to avoid veering off to a completely different course in your life.

Each day is a new day to take steps toward your growth, and it is an opportunity to begin again. Take each day one step at a time and remember why you started.

Focus on what you want to obtain and get moving. There is no moment like the present to begin again. It is never too late to get back on track.

Chapter 10

Getting to Know the New You

"If you can dream it, you can do it." – Walt Disney

Remember when I said in chapter 3 that this is not really about the weight?

Well, it's not. This is your life, live it fully.

Now it's time to decide what you want next for your life. You've come along on this journey for a reason as we've discussed during this entire book.

You've done a lot of work on yourself and now you want to reap the rewards!

This whole time I hope you've been digging deep, practicing your new tools of awareness, and been getting to know the new you.

For a long, long time, it's always been about the weight, and now it's not.

So, in this chapter, I want you to think about what you REALLY, REALLY want for the next chapter in your life, for the thinner version of you.

What have you always wanted to accomplish?

What have you always wanted to do?

What are your dreams?

What excites you?

What do you get to do now that you've lost the weight?

And, even if you haven't hit goal yet, that's OK. The point here is that for most of your life (like mine) you've spent your time thinking, feeling, planning, dreaming, and/or worrying about food, what and when you'll eat, how much, and then how to burn it off.

You know, and I know, that those old behaviors were not truly about living, but about obsession and emotional comfort.

Now that we're working on those issues, it's important to look forward to the future, to the new life that you have before you.

The path outlined in this book is designed to help you work WITH food, and to build new behavioral and mental pathways to help encourage you to live BEYOND the food.

If this is still a struggle, I strongly encourage you to reach out to a mental health professional specializing in eating disorders, bariatric or obesity-related issues.

This book is not a one size fits all, and some people just need more intimate help one-on-one to help them dig deeper into their emotions, mind, or past to deal with other issues that may be the root of the problem.

This part of the process can be troublesome and daunting because many people avoid doing the work necessary to get to know the NEW you.

The truth is while you haven't changed, you have completely changed at the same time. You look different on the outside and you may notice that you'll get treated differently and either people will look at you more, or look at you less.

This is just one example of how you'll experience the world differently.

In other ways you'll have opportunities that you didn't have before. You'll get to do things that you would not have otherwise been able to do. Losing the weight is the first step in living the life of your dreams. Now, you get to go and do all the things you've always wanted to do.

Have you ever wondered why people have bariatric surgery and then go on to be triathletes?

Did they always want to be triathletes?

Most likely, no.

However, when your body changes and you start to move more, it feels good to continue to move more, and more, and more. It's an easy step for many people to become an athlete after experiencing cabin fever for many years, not wanting to leave the house, or experiencing shame when it comes to moving or walking in public.

This chapter is about exploring who you are and what you've always wanted to do and accomplish.

One of my clients came into my office recently and told me that she always wanted to bungee jump. She shared this as though she was telling me something very secretive and was very hesitant to share it.

When I asked her why this was such a big secret, she shared that when she was 482 lb., she could not see herself bungee jumping because she knew she would not have the ability to brace herself if she needed to.

Another thing she shared was that when she told her family, they made some horrible jokes that made her feel self-conscious, which made her keep even more of her dreams hidden away.

People can be cruel and hurtful to individuals with obesity and, therefore, many obese individuals keep their hopes and dreams locked away.

They may hide their true dreams and ambitions believing that "there's no way I could get that job," or "there's no way that woman/man would ever look at me romantically," or "how could someone like me ever run a 5K?"

This is the point at which we work to shift your thinking through doing things differently. It's not just about how you feel or how you think, but also in how you behave. Of course, you'll want to take a deeper look at what you really want for your life, so that you gain clarity in that area.

Another good point to note here is that many people know what they do NOT want more often than what they DO want. We want to avoid talking about what you don't want, and we want to get clear on what you DO want.

So, if you need to make a list of things that you do NOT want, to help you get clear on what you DO want, go ahead and do that.

However, for the exercises in this chapter, start to daydream and think about all the things you'd like to be, do, or have in your life so you can get super clear about what they are and how you can achieve them.

This is an opportunity to explore things you've always wanted to do and create the life you've always dreamed of. Using this chapter can also help you outline your goals as you reach your weight loss goals, you will be closer to achieving many other things in life that you may not have been physically able to do prior to weight loss surgery.

How awesome is that?

Acting "as if" is a great way to develop these skills.

How would you behave at work if you knew you could snag that senior executive management position with ease?

How would you feel if you could walk up to that hot guy in the bar and strike up a friendly conversation with ease?

How would you feel if you could run a 5K without feeling the aches and pains in your joints, or need to stop for air in the middle?

When you start to take action on who you want to be by stepping into that role, by acting and behaving in that manner, you begin to build the expectation that you WILL get there, and you'll notice a shift in your energy.

My client Megan always wanted to go skydiving. However, she was absolutely frightened at the idea of jumping out of a plane at 450 lb. She knew her leg muscles weren't strong and often thought to herself that no one would ever allow her up in the plane, with it being a risk due to her weight.

In our sessions after her weight loss surgery, we began conducting visualizations of Megan jumping out of the plane at a weight she was confident she would be allowed to jump at. Every time she did this exercise, she would get giddy. It took Megan about 16 months to get to the weight where she felt confident she would be able to skydive, and she took to the skies.

She returned to tell me that it was one of the happiest days of her life and that having the goal of skydiving helped her stay on track while also fulfilling a lifelong dream of hers.

Each of these goals can have multiple layers, they do not need to serve a single purpose of "when I get to this weight, then I can _____" (fill in the blank).

Conversely, your goals may help you stay on track knowing that if you do not stay on track, you'll never get to do whatever is you've set your mind to do.

Or, it could be the goal itself that helps you get to the next level in your life so that you can reach the next goal, and the next one, and the next one.

There is no limit, and the only limits we have are the ones we create in our minds. So, dream big, and start making a list of all the things you'd like to achieve at any given weight, and start moving toward them.

Building Your Bucket List

"The future belongs to those who believe in the beauty of their dreams." – Eleanor Roosevelt

This is your opportunity to get real with yourself. You've been given a second chance, a new lease on life, and so what are you going to do with it?

Are you planning on climbing Everest?

Will you become a parent?

Will you go back to school, so you can get the degree and land the dream job?

Or maybe you are going straight for the dream job?

Are you nearing retirement and have plans to travel the world?

What is it that you'd like to be, do, and have in your life after weight loss surgery?

One of my favorite exercises in coaching is called the BE – DO – HAVE and we will write exactly that.

Take out your notebook or journal and write one of the following on the top of three sheets of paper.

On one you'll write: Who do I want to BE?

One the next you'll write: What do I want to DO?

On the third, you'll write: What do I desire to HAVE?

Then start creating your lists of who you want to be, what you want to do, and what you'd like to have in your life following bariatric surgery. There is no limit, and you can write these lists in multiple ways so that you gain insight into your desires.

When I do this with clients, I ask people to get free and wild with their desires. Also, be mindful that your "have" list can be things, people, or situations that you'd like in your life.

Use these as your guide and build your own!

"BE" examples

I want to be a woman who is secure in herself.

I want to be a doctor.

I want to be a triathlete.

I want to be a mentor to others.

"DO" examples

I want to go back to school and pursue that nursing degree.

I want to go for daily walks with my husband.

I want to go after that promotion at work.

I want to travel to Hawaii with my girlfriends.

I want to climb Machu Picchu.

<u>"HAVE" examples</u>

I want to have a happy relationship with my husband.

I'd like to have a better relationship with my colleagues at work.

I want to have a sports car that is reflective of my personality.

I want to have a baby.

I want to have my own business.

See how they can vary from things to situations, to relationships, to your own personal life?

Get creative and revisit this list every few months to see what you have achieved, and to see what has changed in your desires. It may surprise you that you may or may not want the same things you thought about a few months ago.

You can get as simple or as extravagant with this list as you like. It gets you to start thinking about all the things you'd like to create in your life and getting you thinking of your NEW life, which is awesome!

Affirming Your Dreams

Your life is important. Having bariatric surgery was just the first step in getting your life back. Addressing the lifestyle change was another portion, and now it's time for you to step into the life you desire. Affirming your dreams is more than just creating affirmations that are whimsical or airy-fairy.

It's about creating your dreams first within your mind, and then into your reality by taking steps toward your goals. Each chapter before this one has given you guidance in achieving your goals and guiding you to take flight toward your dreams. Whether you are at goal weight yet or not, it's time to start the systematic belief that you will arrive by affirming that you already have arrived.

When you feel the feelings of achieving all that you want, your mindset and attitude shift with it. Also, by affirming what you desire, this helps you gain perspective on what you truly want and how you'd like to feel, so that each action you take after it, is intentional.

For example, if you were to say, "I love how I feel so awesome and in charge of my eating around food at parties" while using visualizations of having a great time, as discussed in an earlier chapter, you would be prepared to go to the party feeling calmer and in charge. Additionally, you'll likely feel excited to achieve that. It's more than an affirmation, it's a goal statement.

Use these affirming statements to tap into how you want to feel in multiple areas of your life and see what comes up for you. This is a great way to dive into another area of your psyche to see what you'd like to achieve, overcome, conquer, or complete in your life.

Also, be aware that some of these examples might not be directly weight-related; however, we know that obesity takes a toll on self-esteem and feeling "good enough" in a variety of roles in one's life.

Therefore, some of the examples above below are reflected in both the external physical changes and the inner mindset work completed to feel confident, successful, and worthy of greatness in one's own life. Also, the examples below are suggestions – feel free to make your own that reflect how you want to feel in your own life.

❖ **Career/Work Dreams**

I am confident in my abilities at work.

I am excited to be seen at work because I add value there.

I am excited to take on new roles and responsibilities at work because I can physically take them on, which is amazing!

I am excited to ask for a raise because I know I'm worthy and deserving of it and feel confident in my abilities.

❖ **Personal Lifestyle Dreams**

I love how easy it is for me to get up and move around.

I love how easy my clothes fit me.

I love how I look in the mirror.

I love how I feel in my body.

❖ **Fitness / Marathon / 5K Goals / Dreams**

I see myself crossing the finish line at _____.

Crossing the finish line makes me feel _____.

Being fit makes me feel _____.

I love how my body feels when I work out.

I love that I can lift 50 lb. easily and effortlessly.

I love how I can walk a 5K with ease, and I also have fun doing it.

I love how I can walk/run easily without pain.

❖ Travel Dreams

I love how I fit in the airline seat perfectly without a seatbelt extender.

I love how I can comfortably fly across the world without worrying about blood clots, bothering someone to move, having trouble getting out of my seat, without needing help.

I love how I can climb the stairs of Machu Picchu without feeling out of breath.

❖ Eating Dreams

I love how I can go to a restaurant and not feel the need to order 10 things.

I love how I can go to a restaurant and push away food while feeling completely satiated.

I love how I can go out with friends, make healthy choices and feel good about myself.

I love how I can go to parties and stick with my eating plan successfully.

❖ Relationship Dreams

I love how my husband/wife looks at me.

I love dating a person who values me for who I am.

I love having people in my life who support me and encourage me to be a better person.

I love surrounding myself with positive people.

All my relationships are amazing.

Repeat these exercises every few months to see what you've accomplished, what goals you've reached, and what you'd like to change or add to your goals and dreams.

In these exercises, you are stretching who you are and who you've known yourself to be. You've been on autopilot thinking and living for far too long. I hope that each of these exercises serves you to think bigger and better in terms of your life after bariatric surgery and continues to help you build your motivation and momentum toward success.

It is recommended that you come back to this chapter and utilize these exercises every couple of months to see what has changed and what you've already improved on or achieved in your life. While each person has their own list of goals, the more you achieve, the more goals you'll create for yourself. Just remember that there is no limit, only the ones that you create in your mind.

Remember, this is a process, your process, and true lifestyle change.

I hope this book serves you well and that you go back to comb over the chapters as they guide you to stay on track. It was from my own pain, my own growth, and my own passion to serve others that this book has been born.

I wrote this hoping that this reaches each person who has struggled with the pain of obesity in the hope that you utilize the tools in this book so that you shift your mindset to reach your ultimate goal after weight loss surgery: bariatric mindset success. If you think this will help someone, please share it!

As you continue your journey, if you'd like additional support, feel free to join our free private online Facebook group: Bariatric Mindset Mavens

www.facebook.com/groups/bariatricmindset

To track your new habits and behaviors, grab the new *Bariatric Mindset Success Accountability Journal*, available in 3-month and 6-month formats on Amazon. It will be an amazing asset to your progress! I have also created a *Rediscover You Journal* and *Color Your Confidence Coloring Book* to aid you on your journey.

Check out my newest book, *Release Your Regain*, also available on Amazon.

Also, for more information on upcoming book releases, check out www.bariatricmindset.com and join our mailing list for additional offers, freebies, blogs, and support on your bariatric mindset success journey.

Helping you to live your best life and keep the weight off after weight loss surgery, Bariatric Mindset is your partner in success.

Appendices

Appendix A:

Bariatric Mindset – High-Protein Food List – Grams of Each Listed

- **Beef**
  - Hamburger patty, 4 oz. – 28 g protein
  - Steak, 6 oz. – 42 g protein
  - Filet Mignon, 3 oz. – 22 g protein
  - Most cuts of beef – 7 g of protein per ounce
  - Deli lunch meat – Boars Head London Broil (Beef), 2 oz. – 12 g protein
- **Chicken**
  - Chicken breast, 3.5 oz. – 30 g protein
  - Chicken thigh – 10 g (for average size)
  - Drumstick – 11 g
  - Wing – 6 g
  - Chicken meat, cooked, 4 oz. – 35 g
  - Costco Rotisserie Chicken Meat (prepared), 3 oz. – 19 g
  - Lunch meat –
    - Boars Head Maple Glazed Honey Coated Turkey, 2 oz. – 14 g
    - Boars Head Teriyaki Chicken (2 oz.) – 12 g
- **Seafood/Fish**
  - Most fish steaks or fish fillets are about 18–23 g of protein for 3.5 oz. cooked, or 6 g per ounce uncooked (salmon, halibut, grouper, mahi-mahi, etc.)
  - Tuna, 6 oz. can – 40 g of protein

- o Tuna pouches – 2.6 oz. = 14 g protein, flavors available in StarKist brand: Ranch, Lemon Pepper, Hickory Smoked, Sweet & Spicy, Bacon Ranch, Honey BBQ
- o Shrimp, 3 oz. – 11.6 g protein
- o Stone Crab Claws – 3 claws, 4 oz. – 15 g
- o King Crabmeat cooked, 3 oz. – 16 g
- o Lobster, 1 cup – 28 g protein
- o Oyster, 3 oz. – 4.4 g protein
- o Scallops, 1 cup – 24 g protein
- o Clams, 3 oz. – 12.5 g protein
- **Pork**
  - o Pork chop, average – 22 g protein
  - o Pork loin or tenderloin, 4 oz. – 29 g
  - o Pork ribs, 3 oz. – 19 g protein
  - o Ham, 3 oz. – 19 g
  - o Ground pork, 1 oz. raw – 5 g; 3 oz. cooked – 22 g
  - o Bacon, 1 slice – 3 g
  - o Canadian-style bacon (back bacon), slice – 5–6 g
  - o Boars Head Maple Glazed Honey Coated Ham, 2 oz. – 10 g
- **Eggs and Dairy**
  - o Egg, large – 6 g protein
  - o Milk, 1 cup – 8 g
  - o Cottage cheese, ½ cup – 15 g
  - o Yogurt, 1 cup – usually 8–15 g, check label
  - o Greek yogurt, 1 cup – usually 21–23 g, check label
  - o Soft cheeses (mozzarella, Brie, Camembert) – 6 g per oz.
  - o Medium cheeses (Colby Jack, Cheddar, Swiss) – 7 or 8 g per oz.
  - o Hard cheeses (Parmesan) – 10 g per oz.
- **Beans (including soy)**
  - o Tofu, ½ cup – 20 g protein

- o Tofu, 1 oz. – 2.3 g
- o Soy milk, 1 cup – 6–10 g
- o Most beans (black, pinto, lentils, chickpeas, etc.) about 7–10 g protein per half cup of cooked beans
- o Shelled soybeans , ½ cup cooked – 14 g protein
- o Split peas, ½ cup cooked – 8 g
- **Nuts and Seeds**
  - o Peanut butter, 2 tablespoons – 8 g protein
  - o Almonds, ¼ cup – 8 g
  - o Peanuts, ¼ cup – 9 g
  - o Cashews, ¼ cup – 5 g
  - o Pecans, ¼ cup – 2.5 g
  - o Sunflower seeds, ¼ cup – 6 g
  - o Pumpkin seeds, ¼ cup – 8 g
  - o Flax seeds – ¼ cup – 8 g
- **Other Protein Sources**
  - o Quest Nutrition Protein Bars – 20 g–22 g per bar
  - o Unjury Whey Isolate Protein Powder One scoop – 20 g protein, or ready-to-drink options
  - o MuscleTech Nitro-Tech Protein Powder, one scoop – 30 g protein
  - o Orgain, Organic Plant Based Protein Powder – 21 g protein

Appendix B:

Feelings Chart		OPTIMISTIC	HOPEFUL, INSPIRED
	Happy	TRUSTING	SENSITIVE, INTIMATE
		PEACEFUL	LOVING, THANKFUL
		POWERFUL	COURAGEOUS, CREATIVE
		ACCEPTED	RESPECTED, VALUED
		PROUD	SUCCESSFUL, CONFIDENT, FULFILLED
		INTERESTED	CURIOUS, INQUISITIVE
		CONTENT	FREE, JOYFUL
		PLAYFUL	AMUSED, CHEEKY
	Surprised	EXCITED	EAGER, ENERGETIC
		AMAZED	ASTONISHED, AWE
		CONFUSED	DISILLUSIONED, PERPLEXED
		STARTLED	SHOCKED, DISMAYED
	Bad	TIRED	SLEEPY, UNFOCUSED, LAZY
		STRESSED	OVERWHELMED, OUT OF CONTROL
		BUSY	PRESSURED, RUSHED
		BORED	INDIFFERENT, APATHETIC
	Fearful	THREATENED	NERVOUS, EXPOSED
		REJECTED	EXCLUDED, PERSECUTED
		WEAK	WORTHLESS, INSIGNIFICANT
		INSECURE	INADEQUATE, CYNICAL
		ANXIOUS	OVERWHELMED, WORRIED
		SCARED	HELPLESS, FRIGHTENED
	Angry	CRITICAL	SKEPTICAL, DISMISSIVE
		DISTANT	WITHDRAWN, NUMB
		FRUSTRATED	INFURIATED, ANNOYED
		AGGRESSIVE	PROVOKED, HOSTILE
		MAD	FURIOUS, JEALOUS
		BITTER	INDIGNANT, VIOLATED
		HUMILIATED	DISRESPECTED, RIDICULED
		LET DOWN	BETRAYED, RESENTFUL
	Disgusted	REPELLED	HORRIFIED, HESITANT
		AWFUL	NAUSEATED, DETESTABLE
		DISAPPOINTED	APPALLED, REVOLTED
		DISAPPROVING	JUDGMENTAL, OFFENDED
	Sad	HURT	EMBARRASSED, DISAPPOINTED
		DEPRESSED	EMPTY, INFERIOR
		GUILTY	ASHAMED, REMORSEFUL
		DESPAIR	GRIEF, POWERLESS
		VULNERABLE	VICTIMIZED, FRAGILE
		LONELY	ISOLATED, ABANDONED

Bibliography

ACEP. (2017). CEP and EFT Defined – Association for Comprehensive Energy Psychology, www.energypsych.org/?ComparingEFTandCEP.

Benedict, Christian (2014). "The fat mass and obesity-associated gene (FTO) is linked to higher plasma levels of the hunger hormone ghrelin and lower serum levels of the satiety hormone leptin in older adults." Diabetes (New York, N.Y.) (0012-1797), 63 (11), p. 3955.

Canfield, J., & Switzer, J. (2015). The success principles: How to get from where you are to where you want to be. New York: William Morrow.

Covey, S. R. (1998). The 7 habits of highly effective people. Provo, UT: Franklin Covey.

Hardy, D. (2013). The compound effect: Multiplying your success, one simple step at a time. Philadelphia: Da Capo Press, Perseus Books Group.

Hensrud, M. D. (2015, April 16). Why skipping sleep leads to weight gain. Retrieved from http://www.mayoclinic.org/healthy-lifestyle/adult-health/expert-answers/sleep-and-weight-gain/faq-20058198

How many hours of sleep do you need? (2016, April 06). Retrieved from http://www.mayoclinic.org/healthy-lifestyle/adult-health/expert-answers/how-many-hours-of-sleep-are-enough/faq-20057898

Klaczynski, P. A., Goold, K. W., & Mudry, J. J. (2004). Culture, Obesity Stereotypes, Self-Esteem, and the Thin Ideal: A Social Identity Perspective. Journal of Youth and Adolescence, 33(4), 307–317. doi:10.1023/b:joyo.0000032639.71472.19

Mans, E., Serra-Prat, M., Palomera, E., Sunol, X., & Clave, P. (2015). Sleeve gastrectomy effects on hunger, satiation, and gastrointestinal hormone and motility responses after a liquid meal test. American Journal of Clinical Nutrition, 102(3), 540–547. doi:10.3945/ajcn.114.104307

McCallie, M. S., Blum, C. M., & Hood, C. J. (2006). Progressive muscle relaxation. Journal of Human Behavior in the Social Environment, 13(3), 51–66.

Mcgrice, M., & Paul, K. D. (2015). Interventions to improve long-term weight loss in patients following bariatric surgery: Challenges and solutions. Diabetes, Metabolic Syndrome and Obesity: Targets and Therapy, 263. doi:10.2147/dmso.s57054

Mirza, N. M., Mackey, E. R., Armstrong, B., Jaramillo, A., & Palmer, M. M. (2011). Correlates of self-worth and body size dissatisfaction among obese Latino youth. Body Image, 8(2), 173–178. doi:10.1016/j.bodyim.2010.12.002

Neff, K. D. (2003). The Development and Validation of a Scale to Measure Self-Compassion. Self and Identity, 2(3), 223–250. doi:10.1080/1529886030902

Neff, K. (2017). What Self-Compassion is Not: Self-esteem, self-pity, indulgence. Retrieved from http://self-compassion.org/what-self-compassion-is-not-2

Neff, K. (2017). Definition and Three Elements of Self Compassion | Kristin Neff. Retrieved from http://self-compassion.org/the-three-elements-of-self-compassion-2/

Odom, J., Zalesin, K. C., Washington, T. L., Miller, W. W., Hakmeh, B., Zaremba, D. L., . . . Mccullough, P. A. (2009). Behavioral Predictors of Weight Regain after Bariatric Surgery. Obesity Surgery, 20(3), 349–356. doi:10.1007/s11695-009-9895-6

Orcutt, M., Steffen, K., & Mitchell, J. E. (2017). Eating Disorders and Problematic Eating Behaviors After Bariatric Surgery. Oxford Handbooks Online. doi:10.1093/oxfordhb/9780190620998.013.25

Wing, R. R., & Phelan, S. (2005). Long-term weight loss maintenance. The American Journal of Clinical Nutrition, 82(1), 2225-2255

About the Author

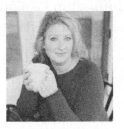

Kristin Lloyd, PhD, has been creating outstanding results for individuals, couples, and organizations for over 15 years as a highly accomplished psychotherapist, transformational mindset mentor, coach, college educator, and consultant.

Through her invigorating and transformative facilitation skills, Kristin has been guiding individuals, couples, and executives to achieve dramatic breakthroughs in mindset and motivation, self-confidence, productivity, commitment, habit-shifting, interpersonal communication, relationship renewal, conflict resolution, stress reduction, and aligning with their soul's purpose as well as reinventing one's future for success.

Kristin's passion for helping people "get out of their own way" led her to work with weight loss surgery patients to shift their mindset after bariatric surgery. As a patient herself, she understands the struggles bariatric patients endure post-op. She works with them to create lasting behavioral/habit changes and emotional adjustments that lead to happy, healthy, and fulfilling lives by keeping the weight off and adjusting to the multitude of lifestyle changes that occur following bariatric surgery.

As a mental health professional, she is passionate about helping people overcome depression, anxiety, self-sabotage, and life stressors so they can achieve balance and sustained success through habit building.

She is also a certified Reiki Master, clinical certified hypnotherapist, an EFT/Energy Psychology Practitioner, speaker, and a prolific writer. Kristin is currently a contributor for The Obesity Action Coalition, Obesity Help, The Huffington Post and The Master Shift. She is also a member of the Obesity Action Coalition.

Follow me on Social Media:

Facebook: www.facebook.com/bariatricmindset

Twitter: @barimindset

Instagram: @bariatricmindset

YouTube: Bariatric Mindset

Made in the USA
Las Vegas, NV
11 September 2023

77370027R00167